DIET

AND

OBESITY

THE ULTIMATE GUIDE TO A HEALTHY DIET FOR THE OBESE AND OVERWEIGHT

DR. STIEN

First Edition 2024

Published by Dr. Stien

Table of Content

Introduction

    Understanding Obesity

    Importance of Diet in Obesity Management

Chapter 1: The Science Behind Obesity

    Body Weight Regulation: How Diet Influences Metabolism

    Role of Genetics and Environment in Obesity

    Inflammation and obesity

Chapter 2: Assessing Your Diet

    Understanding Macronutrients: Carbohydrates, Proteins, Fats

    Micronutrients: Vitamins and Minerals Essential for Health

Chapter 3: Impact of Diet on Weight Management

    Caloric Balance: Energy In vs. Energy Out

    Popular Diets and Their Effectiveness

Chapter 4: Designing a Healthy Eating Plan

    Principles of a Balanced Diet

    Portion Control and Mindful Eating

Chapter 5: Special Considerations in Diet and Obesity

    Childhood Obesity: Causes and Prevention Strategies

    Pregnancy and Obesity: Dietary Recommendations

Obesity and Diabetes

Chapter 6: Psychological Aspects of Eating

Emotional Eating and Stress Management

Strategies for Behavior Change and Sustaining Healthy Habits

Chapter 7: Practical Tips for Grocery Shopping and Meal Preparation

Reading Food Labels: Understanding Nutrient Content

Healthy Cooking Techniques and Recipes

Chapter 8: Physical Activity and its Role in Weight Management

Combining Diet with Exercise: Synergistic Effects

Chapter 9: Long-Term Maintenance of Weight Loss

Strategies for Preventing Weight Regain

Support Systems and Resources for Continued Success

Chapter 10: Myths and Facts about Obesity

Debunking Common Myths

Some Important Facts about Obesity

Chapter 11: Conclusion

Looking Ahead: Future Trends in Diet and Obesity Management

Appendix: Resources and Further Reading

Glossary of Terms

Recommended Websites and Other Books

Introduction

Understanding Obesity

Obesity has become one of the most significant health challenges of our time, impacting millions of people around the globe. More than just an issue of appearance, obesity is defined by the excessive accumulation of body fat, which can seriously affect overall health and well-being. The World Health Organization (WHO) reports that obesity rates have nearly tripled worldwide since 1975, highlighting a global epidemic that urgently needs our attention and action.

What is Obesity?

Obesity is usually determined by body mass index (BMI), which is calculated by dividing a person's weight in kilograms by the square of their height in meters (kg/m^2). A BMI of 30 or higher is considered obese, while a BMI between 25 and 29.9 is classified as overweight. While BMI is a helpful screening tool, it doesn't directly measure body fat percentage or its distribution, both of which are important in assessing the health risks linked to obesity. For instance a body builder may have a BMI of 30 or above but in reality may not be obese. This is because the extra mass is muscle rather than fat.

Why Does Obesity Happen?

The reasons behind obesity are complex and involve a mix of genetic, environmental, behavioral, and societal factors. Genetics can influence how easily someone gains weight, while environmental aspects like sedentary lifestyles and the ready availability of high-calorie foods increase the risk. Additionally, socio-economic factors, cultural attitudes toward food, and psychological factors such as stress eating and emotional triggers all play significant roles in the onset of obesity.

Understanding the causes of obesity is crucial for developing effective prevention and management strategies. By tackling both individual behaviours and societal influences, we can create environments that encourage healthy choices and help reduce the prevalence of obesity-related health issues.

Importance of Diet in Obesity Management

Managing and preventing obesity revolves around diet—it's the cornerstone of weight control and overall health. As stated previously, obesity results from a variety of factors, but they all lead to one fundamental issue: "caloric imbalance." This imbalance occurs when we consume more calories than we burn off, not just through eating any food, but food with high caloric content. These excess calories are then stored as fat, leading to weight gain and eventually, obesity.

To combat obesity, we need to strike a balance between the calories we consume and those we burn. Achieving this balance can be different for everyone, depending on the root cause of the imbalance. In the following chapters, we'll delve into the intricacies of obesity, exploring its main causes and the crucial role diet plays. We'll look at how these factors shape our approach to managing obesity effectively and provide practical tips for achieving and maintaining a healthy weight through smart dietary choices. By equipping ourselves with knowledge and embracing evidence-based strategies, we can tackle obesity head-on, improving our health and quality of life.

Chapter 1: The Science Behind Obesity

Body Weight Regulation: How Diet Influences Metabolism

Imagine your body as a finely tuned machine, constantly working to maintain balance. This balance, or homeostasis, is particularly crucial when it comes to body weight. Every day, your body performs a delicate dance, orchestrating the intake and expenditure of energy to keep your weight stable. But how does it all work? And more importantly, how does your diet play into this complex system?

The Metabolic Orchestra

Think of your metabolism as an orchestra with multiple instruments. Each instrument represents different metabolic processes, and your diet is the conductor. When you consume food, it's like handing sheet music to the musicians. The quality and type of food dictate how each instrument plays, influencing the overall harmony of your metabolic symphony.

Carbohydrates:

When you eat carbs, your body breaks them down into glucose, the primary fuel for your cells. Insulin, a hormone, acts as the conductor, directing glucose into cells for immediate energy or storing it for later use. However, excess glucose can be converted to fat, contributing to weight gain.

Proteins:

Proteins are the building blocks of your body. They are broken down into amino acids, which help repair tissues, build muscle, and produce enzymes. A high-protein diet can boost your metabolism slightly, as it requires more energy to digest and utilise these nutrients, a process known as the thermic effect of food.

Fats:

Dietary fats are essential for absorbing vitamins and protecting organs. They are broken down into fatty acids and glycerol. Unlike carbs and proteins, fats are more calorie-dense, providing a longer-lasting energy source. However, consuming too much fat, especially unhealthy types, can lead to weight gain.

Hormones: The Unsung Heroes

Hormones are the silent messengers in your metabolic orchestra, sending signals that influence hunger, satiety, and energy storage. Let's meet some key players:

<u>Leptin:</u>

Often called the "satiety hormone," leptin is produced by fat cells. It tells your brain when you have enough energy stored and can stop eating. However, in obesity, the brain can become resistant to leptin's signals, leading to overeating.

<u>Ghrelin:</u>

Known as the "hunger hormone," ghrelin is produced in the stomach and signals hunger to the brain. Levels rise before meals and fall after eating. Diets high in processed foods can disrupt this natural rhythm, making you feel hungrier more often.

<u>Insulin:</u>

Beyond its role in glucose management, insulin also affects fat storage. High levels of insulin, often a result of consuming too many refined carbs, can promote fat storage, especially around the abdomen.

So, how does your diet influence this intricate system? It all comes down to the types of foods you eat and how they interact with your metabolism.

Quality Over Quantity:

Not all calories are created equal. Whole foods like fruits, vegetables, lean proteins, and whole grains provide essential nutrients that help your metabolism run smoothly. In contrast, processed foods high in sugar and unhealthy fats can disrupt metabolic processes and lead to weight gain.

Timing Matters:

When you eat can be just as important as what you eat. Irregular eating patterns and late-night snacking can throw off your metabolic rhythm. Consistent meal timing helps regulate hunger hormones and maintains a steady energy supply.

Hydration:

Water is a critical component of metabolism. It helps in the digestion and transportation of nutrients. Staying hydrated can also aid in weight management by promoting satiety and supporting metabolic functions.

<u>Micronutrients:</u>

Vitamins and minerals, though needed in smaller amounts, play significant roles in metabolism. For example, B vitamins are crucial for energy production, while magnesium is involved in over 300 metabolic reactions.

The Bigger Picture

Understanding how diet influences metabolism is a crucial step in managing body weight. It's not just about counting calories; it's about making informed choices that support your body's natural processes. By focusing on nutrient-dense foods, maintaining regular eating patterns, and staying hydrated, you can help your metabolic orchestra play a harmonious symphony, leading to better weight management and overall health.

In the grand scheme of the science of obesity, recognizing the role of diet in regulating metabolism empowers you to take control of your health. So, the next time you sit down for a meal, remember: you're not just eating to satisfy hunger—you're conducting a complex, beautiful symphony that keeps your body in balance.

Role of Genetics and Environment in Obesity

Let's take a journey into the intricate world of body weight regulation, where the interplay between genetics and environment creates a complex tapestry. Imagine your body as a sophisticated machine influenced by its blueprint (genes) and its surroundings (environment). In this section, we'll explore how these factors shape the landscape of obesity.

Genetics: The Blueprint of Your Body

Think of your genes as the master architects of your body, dictating everything from your eye color to your predisposition to certain health conditions, including obesity. But how exactly do genes influence body weight?

The Thrifty Gene Hypothesis:

Historically, humans faced periods of feast and famine. Those with "thrifty genes" were better at storing fat during times of plenty, which helped them survive during lean times. In today's world, where food is abundant, these same genes can predispose individuals to obesity.

<u>Genetic Variants:</u>

Specific genetic variations can affect how your body processes food and stores fat. For example, variations in the FTO gene have been linked to higher body mass index (BMI) and increased risk of obesity. These genetic variants can influence hunger, satiety, and how efficiently your body converts food into energy.

<u>Epigenetics:</u>

Beyond the DNA sequence itself, epigenetics involves changes in gene expression influenced by environmental factors. For instance, poor nutrition or high stress levels can modify how genes are expressed, potentially increasing the risk of obesity.

Environment: The World Around You

While your genes provide the blueprint, your environment supplies the materials and conditions that influence how that blueprint is realised. Let's delve into the various environmental factors that play a role in obesity:

<u>Diet and Nutrition:</u>

The types of food available and consumed can significantly impact body weight. Diets high in processed foods, sugars, and unhealthy fats can lead to weight gain, whereas balanced diets rich in whole foods support healthy weight management.

Physical Activity:

Sedentary lifestyles, often driven by modern conveniences like cars, computers, and televisions, contribute to weight gain. Regular physical activity helps burn calories and maintain a healthy weight.

Socioeconomic Factors:

Access to healthy food options and safe environments for physical activity can be limited by socioeconomic status. Lower-income neighbourhoods might have more fast-food outlets and fewer grocery stores offering fresh produce.

Cultural and Social Influences:

Cultural norms and social practices around food and body image can shape eating habits and perceptions of weight. Social settings often involve food, and societal pressures can influence dietary choices and physical activity levels.

Psychological Factors:

Stress, depression, and other psychological conditions can lead to emotional eating and reduced physical activity, contributing to weight gain. Coping mechanisms often involve food, leading to unhealthy eating patterns.

The Interplay: Genes and Environment Together

The relationship between genetics and environment in obesity is not a simple one; it's a dynamic interplay where each influences the other. Here's how they work together:

Gene-Environment Interaction:

Certain genetic predispositions may only manifest under specific environmental conditions. For example, someone with a genetic tendency to gain weight might only do so in an environment with abundant high-calorie foods and little physical activity.

Environmental Modifications:

While you can't change your genes, you can modify your environment to support healthy weight management. This includes adopting a balanced diet, engaging in regular physical activity, and creating a supportive social network.

Epigenetic Changes:

Environmental factors can lead to epigenetic changes that alter gene expression. For instance, a healthy diet and regular exercise can potentially reverse some of the adverse epigenetic effects associated with poor lifestyle choices.

Navigating the Path to Healthy Weight
Understanding the role of genetics and environment in obesity empowers you to make informed decisions. While your genes may predispose you to certain challenges, your environment and lifestyle choices play a crucial role in determining your body weight.

By creating a supportive environment—through healthy eating, regular physical activity, and stress management—you can positively influence your weight and overall health. Remember, you're not just a passive recipient of your genetic destiny; you have the power to shape your health outcomes through the choices you make every day.

In the grand narrative of obesity, acknowledging the complex dance between genetics and environment allows for a more compassionate and effective approach to weight management. So, as you navigate your own journey, consider both the blueprint and the materials at your disposal, crafting a path towards a healthier, happier you.

Inflammation and obesity

Have you ever wondered why excess weight seems to be linked with so many health problems? It turns out, there's a hidden culprit in the mix: inflammation. But what does inflammation have to do with obesity, and how does your diet come into play? Let's dive into this fascinating connection.

The Inflammatory Cascade

Inflammation is your body's natural response to injury or infection. It's like an internal alarm system, summoning immune cells to defend and repair. In short bursts, inflammation is beneficial. However, when it becomes chronic, it's a different story. Imagine your body being on constant high alert—this is what happens in chronic inflammation, and it's closely tied to obesity.

Fat Cells: More Than Just Storage

Your fat cells, or adipocytes, do more than just store excess energy. They're active players in your body's immune response. Here's how they get involved in inflammation:

<u>Adipokines:</u>

Fat cells release various signaling molecules called adipokines, including leptin and adiponectin. While adiponectin has anti-inflammatory effects, many adipokines promote inflammation.

<u>Cytokines:</u>

Obese individuals often have elevated levels of inflammatory cytokines like TNF-α and IL-6. These cytokines are produced by both fat cells and immune cells within adipose tissue.

The Role of Visceral Fat

Not all fat is created equal. Visceral fat, the kind that wraps around your internal organs, is particularly notorious for fueling inflammation. Unlike subcutaneous fat, which lies just under the skin, visceral fat is more metabolically active and secretes higher levels of inflammatory molecules.

How Diet Fuels the Fire or Not

Your diet plays a significant role in either stoking the flames of inflammation or putting them out. Let's break down the dietary factors involved:

<u>Sugar and Refined Carbohydrates:</u>
High intake of sugar and refined carbs spikes insulin levels and promotes fat storage, particularly visceral fat. This, in turn, increases inflammatory cytokines.

<u>Trans Fats and Saturated Fats:</u>
Found in processed and fried foods, these fats contribute to inflammation. They can trigger the release of inflammatory markers and reduce the production of beneficial anti-inflammatory molecules.

<u>Omega-3 vs. Omega-6 Fatty Acids:</u>
Omega-3 fatty acids (found in fish, flaxseeds, and walnuts) have anti-inflammatory properties. On the other hand, an excess of omega-6 fatty acids (common in vegetable oils and processed foods) can promote inflammation. Balance is key here.

<u>Fiber and Antioxidants:</u>

Diets high in fruits, vegetables, and whole grains provide fiber and antioxidants, which have anti-inflammatory effects. They help reduce oxidative stress and support a healthy gut microbiota, which plays a role in regulating inflammation.

The Vicious Cycle

Chronic inflammation and obesity can create a vicious cycle. As fat cells grow and expand, they produce more inflammatory molecules. This inflammation can impair insulin signaling, leading to insulin resistance and further weight gain. It's a feedback loop that's hard to break but not impossible.

Breaking the Cycle: Dietary Strategies

So, how can you use your diet to combat inflammation and manage obesity? Here are some strategies:

Embrace Whole Foods:

Focus on a diet rich in whole, minimally processed foods. Fruits, vegetables, whole grains, lean proteins, and healthy fats should be your staples.

Limit Sugar and Refined Carbs:

Reducing your intake of sugary drinks, sweets, and refined grains can help lower insulin spikes and reduce fat storage.

Choose Healthy Fats:
Incorporate sources of omega-3 fatty acids into your diet, such as fatty fish (like salmon and mackerel), flaxseeds, and chia seeds. Use olive oil instead of vegetable oils high in omega-6s.

Increase Fiber Intake:
Fiber not only aids in digestion but also supports a healthy gut microbiota, which is crucial for controlling inflammation. Foods high in fiber include beans, lentils, whole grains, fruits, and vegetables.

Stay Hydrated:
Proper hydration supports all bodily functions, including the regulation of inflammation. Aim for plenty of water throughout the day.

Understanding the link between inflammation and obesity empowers you to take control of your health. By making informed dietary choices, you can reduce chronic inflammation, support your metabolism, and manage your weight more effectively. Remember, it's not just about cutting calories; it's about nourishing your body with the right nutrients to break the cycle of inflammation and obesity.

Chapter 2: Assessing Your Diet

Understanding Macronutrients: Carbohydrates, Proteins, Fats

Let's engulf ourselves in the world of macronutrients—those essential building blocks that provide the energy and materials our bodies need to function. Picture macronutrients as the fuel that keeps your engine running smoothly. In this section, we'll explore carbohydrates, proteins, and fats, understanding their roles in your diet and how they influence your body.

Carbohydrates: The Body's Preferred Fuel

Carbohydrates often get a bad rap in diet discussions, but they play a crucial role in your body's energy supply. Think of carbs as the primary fuel for your engine, providing the quick bursts of energy needed for everything from a morning jog to a late-night study session.

Simple vs. Complex Carbs:

Simple carbs, like sugars, are quick to digest and give you a rapid energy boost. However, they can also lead to energy crashes. Complex carbs, found in whole grains, vegetables, and legumes, digest more slowly, providing a steady energy release.

Fiber:

A special type of carbohydrate, fiber is vital for digestive health. It helps regulate blood sugar levels and keeps you feeling full longer. Foods rich in fiber include fruits, vegetables, whole grains, and legumes.

Glycemic Index:

This measures how quickly a carbohydrate-containing food raises your blood sugar. Low-GI foods (like most fruits, vegetables, and whole grains) are better for maintaining stable energy levels and avoiding spikes in blood sugar.

Proteins: The Body's Building Blocks

Proteins are the construction workers of your body, essential for building and repairing tissues, producing enzymes and hormones, and supporting immune function. When you think of proteins, think of strength and structure.

Amino Acids:

Proteins are made up of amino acids, some of which are essential, meaning your body can't produce them, so you must get them from your diet. Animal products (meat, fish, dairy, eggs) and some plant-based foods (quinoa, soy) provide all essential amino acids.

Plant vs. Animal Proteins:

While animal proteins are complete (containing all essential amino acids), you can also get complete protein from plant-based sources by combining foods like beans and rice or hummus and pita.

Muscle Maintenance:

Adequate protein intake is crucial for maintaining muscle mass, especially as you age. It's also important for recovery if you're engaging in regular exercise or strength training.

Fats: The Long-Lasting Fuel

Fats have long been misunderstood, often vilified as the cause of weight gain. However, fats are essential for energy storage, hormone production, and protecting vital organs. They are the long-lasting fuel your body taps into during prolonged activities.

<u>Types of Fat</u>

<u>Saturated Fats:</u>

Found in animal products and some tropical oils, these fats should be consumed in moderation, as excessive intake can raise cholesterol levels.

<u>Unsaturated Fats:</u>

These include monounsaturated and polyunsaturated fats, found in olive oil, avocados, nuts, and fish. They are beneficial for heart health.

<u>Trans Fats:</u>

Artificial trans fats, found in some processed foods, should be avoided as they increase the risk of heart disease.

<u>Omega-3 and Omega-6 Fatty Acids:</u>

These are essential polyunsaturated fats. Omega-3s (found in fish, flaxseeds, walnuts) have anti-inflammatory properties, while omega-6s (found in vegetable oils) need to be balanced with omega-3s to maintain health.

<u>Energy Density:</u>

Fats are more calorie-dense than carbs and proteins, providing 9 calories per gram compared to 4 calories per gram for carbs and proteins. This makes fats an efficient energy source but also easier to overconsume.

Balancing Macronutrients: Creating a Healthy Plate

Understanding how to balance these macronutrients is key to a healthy diet. Here are some practical tips:

Balance and Variety:

Aim for a balanced mix of carbohydrates, proteins, and fats at each meal. Variety ensures you get a wide range of nutrients.

Portion Control:

Pay attention to portion sizes, especially with calorie-dense fats. Use your hand as a guide—your palm for protein, your fist for carbs, and your thumb for fats.

Nutrient Density:

Choose nutrient-dense foods that provide vitamins, minerals, and fiber along with macronutrients. Whole foods like fruits, vegetables, lean meats, fish, nuts, seeds, and whole grains should be staples.

<u>Meal Timing:</u>

Spread your intake of macronutrients throughout the day to maintain energy levels and support metabolism. Regular meals and snacks can prevent overeating and help manage hunger.

Understanding macronutrients empowers you to make informed dietary choices. By recognizing the roles of carbohydrates, proteins, and fats, you can create a balanced diet that supports your energy needs, muscle maintenance, and overall health.

Micronutrients: Vitamins and Minerals Essential for Health

While macronutrients often steal the spotlight in discussions about diet, micronutrients—vitamins and minerals—are the unsung heroes that keep your body running smoothly. Think of them as the nuts and bolts of a well-oiled machine, ensuring everything functions as it should. In this section, we'll explore the essential vitamins and minerals that play critical roles in your health and how you can ensure you're getting enough of them in your diet.

Vitamins: The Body's Spark Plugs

Vitamins are organic compounds that your body needs in small amounts for a variety of functions. They act as catalysts in numerous biochemical reactions, helping to release energy from food, build proteins and cells, and regulate your metabolism. Here's a closer look at some key vitamins:

Vitamin A:

Essential for vision, immune function, and skin health. It's found in foods like carrots, sweet potatoes, and leafy greens. Think of it as the vitamin that helps you see in the dark and keeps your defenses strong.

B Vitamins:

This group includes B1 (thiamine), B2 (riboflavin), B3 (niacin), B5 (pantothenic acid), B6 (pyridoxine), B7 (biotin), B9 (folate), and B12 (cobalamin). They play crucial roles in energy production, red blood cell formation, and neurological function. Whole grains, meat, eggs, and legumes are rich sources. Imagine B vitamins as the crew that keeps your energy levels up and your brain firing on all cylinders.

Vitamin C:

Known for its role in immune health, vitamin C is also vital for collagen production, wound healing, and as an antioxidant. Citrus fruits, strawberries, bell peppers, and broccoli are excellent sources. Think of vitamin C as your body's repairman, fixing and maintaining tissues.

Vitamin D:

Essential for calcium absorption and bone health, vitamin D is also important for immune function. Your body can produce it when exposed to sunlight, but it's also found in fortified foods and fatty fish. Picture vitamin D as the key that unlocks calcium's benefits for your bones.

Vitamin E:

Acts as a powerful antioxidant, protecting cells from damage. It's found in nuts, seeds, and green leafy vegetables. Vitamin E is like a shield for your cells, defending against oxidative stress.

Vitamin K:

Necessary for blood clotting and bone health. Green leafy vegetables like spinach and kale are rich in vitamin K.

Imagine vitamin K as the clotting factor that stops you from bleeding too much when you get a cut.

Minerals: The Building Blocks

Minerals are inorganic elements that your body needs for various functions, including building bones, making hormones, and regulating heartbeat. Here are some essential minerals:

Calcium:

Vital for strong bones and teeth, muscle function, and nerve signalling. Dairy products, fortified plant milks, and leafy greens are good sources. Calcium is the brick and mortar for your skeletal structure.

Iron:

Crucial for making haemoglobin, the protein in red blood cells that carries oxygen throughout your body. Iron is found in red meat, beans, lentils, and fortified cereals. Think of iron as the oxygen transporter that keeps your body energized.

Magnesium:

Involved in over 300 biochemical reactions, including energy production, muscle contractions, and nerve function. Nuts, seeds, whole grains, and green leafy vegetables are rich in magnesium. Magnesium is the multitasker that supports numerous vital functions.

Potassium:

Helps maintain fluid balance, muscle contractions, and nerve signals. Bananas, potatoes, and legumes are good sources. Potassium is the regulator that ensures your cells stay hydrated and your heart beats properly.

Zinc:

Important for immune function, wound healing, and DNA synthesis. Meat, shellfish, legumes, and seeds are rich in zinc. Zinc is like the repairman that helps your body heal and grow.

Selenium:

Acts as an antioxidant and supports thyroid function. Brazil nuts, seafood, and eggs are good sources. Selenium is the protector, defending your cells from damage.

Balancing Your Micronutrient Intake

Ensuring you get enough vitamins and minerals doesn't have to be complicated. Here are some tips to help you maintain a balanced intake:

Eat a Variety of Foods:

A diverse diet rich in fruits, vegetables, whole grains, lean proteins, and healthy fats ensures you get a wide range of micronutrients.

Focus on Whole Foods:

Whole, unprocessed foods are typically more nutrient-dense than their processed counterparts.

Watch for Deficiencies:

Certain populations, such as vegetarians, vegans, pregnant women, and the elderly, may need to pay extra attention to their intake of specific vitamins and minerals, such as B12, iron, and calcium.

Consider Supplements:

If you have trouble getting enough micronutrients from food alone, supplements can help. However, it's best to consult with a healthcare provider before starting any new supplement regimen.

Conclusion: The Micronutrient Blueprint

Understanding the role of vitamins and minerals in your diet is crucial for maintaining overall health. These micronutrients work behind the scenes, ensuring your body functions optimally. By focusing on a balanced and varied diet, you can provide your body with the essential tools it needs to stay healthy and vibrant.

Chapter 3: Impact of Diet on Weight Management

Caloric Balance: Energy In vs. Energy Out

Ever wonder why some people seem to eat whatever they want and never gain a pound, while others struggle with their weight despite careful dieting? The answer lies in the concept of caloric balance, a fundamental principle of weight management. Understanding the delicate balance between the calories you consume (energy in) and the calories you burn (energy out) is key to managing your weight effectively.

The Basics of Caloric Balance

Caloric balance is the relationship between the amount of energy you take in through food and drink and the amount of energy you expend through basic bodily functions and physical activity. Let's break it down:

<u>Energy In:</u>

This is the total number of calories you consume from foods and beverages. Every morsel you eat and every sip you take contributes to your energy intake.

<u>Energy Out:</u>

This includes the calories your body uses for basic metabolic functions (basal metabolic rate or BMR), physical activity, and the process of digesting food (thermogenesis).

Basal Metabolic Rate (BMR): Your Body's Baseline

Your BMR is the number of calories your body needs to maintain basic physiological functions while at rest, such as breathing, circulation, and cell production. Think of it as the energy cost of keeping your body's lights on. Factors influencing BMR include:

<u>Age:</u>

BMR tends to decrease with age.

<u>Gender:</u>

Men typically have a higher BMR than women due to higher muscle mass.

Body Composition:

More muscle mass increases BMR since muscle burns more calories at rest than fat.

Genetics:

Some people naturally have a higher or lower BMR.

Physical Activity: The Calorie Burner

Physical activity accounts for the calories you burn beyond your BMR. This includes all forms of movement, from structured exercise like running or lifting weights to everyday activities like walking, cleaning, and even fidgeting. The more active you are, the more calories you burn.

Exercise:

Regular workouts can significantly boost your energy expenditure.

Non-Exercise Activity Thermogenesis (NEAT):

This includes all the calories burned from activities other than exercise, like taking the stairs, gardening, or playing with your kids.

Thermic Effect of Food (TEF): The Hidden Cost

Digesting, absorbing, and metabolising food also requires energy, known as the thermic effect of food. Different macronutrients have varying TEF:

<u>Protein:</u>

Has the highest TEF, meaning it takes more energy to digest and process protein than carbs or fats.

<u>Carbohydrates:</u>

Have a moderate TEF.

<u>Fats:</u>

Have the lowest TEF.

Achieving Caloric Balance

Achieving and maintaining a healthy weight is all about balancing energy in with energy out:

<u>Caloric Surplus:</u>

Consuming more calories than you burn leads to weight gain. Your body stores the excess energy as fat.

Caloric Deficit:

Burning more calories than you consume leads to weight loss. Your body taps into stored fat for energy.

Caloric Balance:

Consuming and burning an equal number of calories maintains your current weight.

Practical Tips for Managing Caloric Balance

Track Your Intake:

Keeping a food diary or using an app can help you become more aware of how many calories you're consuming.

Stay Active:

Incorporate physical activity into your daily routine. Aim for a mix of aerobic exercise and strength training for optimal results.

Mind Your Portions:

Pay attention to portion sizes to avoid overeating, especially with high-calorie foods.

<u>Choose Nutrient-Dense Foods:</u>

Opt for foods that provide vitamins, minerals, and fiber along with calories. Think fruits, vegetables, whole grains, lean proteins, and healthy fats.

<u>Listen to Your Body:</u>

Pay attention to hunger and fullness cues. Eating mindfully can help you avoid consuming unnecessary calories.

The Individual Difference

It's important to recognize that everyone's caloric balance is unique. Factors like genetics, metabolism, and lifestyle all play a role. What works for one person might not work for another, so finding a balance that suits your body and lifestyle is very important.

Understanding caloric balance is like understanding the fundamentals of financial budgeting. Just as you balance your income and expenses to manage your finances, you balance your calorie intake and expenditure to manage your weight. By making informed choices about what you eat and how you move, you can achieve a healthy caloric balance that supports your weight management goals.

Popular Diets and Their Effectiveness

The world of dieting can feel like navigating a maze. With so many popular diets out there, each promising transformative results, it can be challenging to know which path to take. In this section, we'll explore some of the most well-known diets, breaking down their principles, potential benefits, and effectiveness. Let's dive into this diet smorgasbord and see what each has to offer.

The Keto Diet: High Fat, Low Carb

The ketogenic diet, or keto for short, is a high-fat, low-carbohydrate eating plan that aims to shift your body into a state of ketosis. In ketosis, your body burns fat for fuel instead of carbohydrates.

<u>Principles:</u>

The keto diet typically consists of 70-80% fat, 10-20% protein, and 5-10% carbohydrates. By drastically reducing carbs, your body starts to use fat as its primary energy source.

Benefits:

Many people experience rapid weight loss, reduced hunger, and improved mental clarity. It's also been shown to help manage conditions like epilepsy, type 2 diabetes, and metabolic syndrome.

Effectiveness:

The keto diet can be effective for short-term weight loss and improving certain health markers. However, it may be challenging to maintain long-term due to its restrictive nature. Additionally, some people may experience the "keto flu" during the initial adaptation period.

The Mediterranean Diet: A Heart-Healthy Choice
The Mediterranean diet is inspired by the traditional eating patterns of countries bordering the Mediterranean Sea. It emphasizes whole foods, healthy fats, and a balanced approach to eating.

Principles:

This diet focuses on fruits, vegetables, whole grains, legumes, nuts, and seeds. Olive oil is the primary fat source, with moderate consumption of fish, poultry, and dairy, and limited red meat and sweets.

<u>Benefits:</u>

Known for its heart-health benefits, the Mediterranean diet is linked to reduced risks of cardiovascular disease, certain cancers, and improved cognitive function. It also promotes weight loss and maintenance.

<u>Effectiveness:</u>

The Mediterranean diet is highly regarded for its sustainability and overall health benefits. It's less about strict rules and more about a lifestyle that emphasizes balanced eating and enjoyment of food.

The Paleo Diet: Eating Like Our Ancestors

The paleo diet, or "caveman diet," is based on the idea that we should eat like our prehistoric ancestors, focusing on whole, unprocessed foods.

<u>Principles:</u>

The paleo diet includes lean meats, fish, fruits, vegetables, nuts, and seeds while excluding dairy, grains, legumes, and processed foods.

<u>Benefits:</u>

Advocates claim the paleo diet can lead to weight loss, improved energy levels, and better blood sugar control. It emphasizes nutrient-dense foods and avoids processed ingredients.

<u>Effectiveness:</u>

While the paleo diet can be effective for weight loss and improving health markers, its exclusion of entire food groups (like grains and legumes) can make it difficult to follow long-term and may lead to nutrient deficiencies if not carefully managed.

The Vegan Diet: Plant-Based Power

The vegan diet excludes all animal products, including meat, dairy, eggs, and even honey. It's rooted in ethical, environmental, and health considerations.

<u>Principles:</u>

A vegan diet focuses on fruits, vegetables, grains, legumes, nuts, and seeds. It emphasizes whole, plant-based foods and avoids all forms of animal exploitation.

<u>Benefits:</u>

Veganism is associated with lower risks of heart disease, hypertension, type 2 diabetes, and certain cancers. It can also lead to weight loss due to its high fiber and low-calorie nature.

<u>Effectiveness:</u>

A well-planned vegan diet can be highly effective for weight loss and overall health. However, it requires careful planning to ensure adequate intake of nutrients like vitamin B12, iron, calcium, and omega-3 fatty acids.

The Intermittent Fasting (IF) Approach: Timing Is Everything

Intermittent fasting isn't a diet in the traditional sense but a pattern of eating that cycles between periods of fasting and eating.

<u>Principles:</u>

Common methods include the 16/8 method (16 hours of fasting, 8 hours of eating), the 5:2 method (eating normally for 5 days, reducing calorie intake to 500-600 calories for 2 days), and the eat-stop-eat method (24-hour fast once or twice a week).

<u>Benefits:</u>

IF can help with weight loss, improved metabolic health, and enhanced cellular repair processes. It may also simplify meal planning and reduce the risk of chronic diseases.

<u>Effectiveness:</u>

Many people find IF effective for weight management and metabolic health. However, it's not suitable for everyone, particularly those with a history of eating disorders or certain medical conditions.

The Low-Carb Diet: Cutting Down on Carbs

Low-carb diets, such as the Atkins diet, focus on reducing carbohydrate intake and increasing protein and fat consumption.

<u>Principles:</u>

These diets limit foods high in carbohydrates, like grains, legumes, fruits, and starchy vegetables, while encouraging meat, fish, eggs, dairy, and non-starchy vegetables.

<u>Benefits:</u>

Low-carb diets can lead to significant weight loss, reduced hunger, and better blood sugar control. They're also effective for short-term weight loss and improving certain health markers.

<u>Effectiveness:</u>

While low-carb diets can be effective for weight loss and health improvements, they may not be sustainable for everyone and can sometimes lead to nutrient imbalances.

Navigating the world of diets can be overwhelming, but the key is finding an approach that works for you—one that fits your lifestyle, preferences, and health goals. Each of these popular diets has its own set of principles, benefits, and challenges. What's most important is choosing a plan you can stick with and that promotes overall health and well-being.

Chapter 4: Designing a Healthy Eating Plan

Principles of a Balanced Diet

When it comes to designing a healthy eating plan, the phrase "balanced diet" often comes up. But what does it really mean to have a balanced diet? It's not just about eating the right amount of food, but also about getting the right nutrients in the right proportions. Let's delve into the principles of a balanced diet and how you can incorporate them into your daily life to achieve optimal health and weight management.

Variety: The Spice of Life

One of the key principles of a balanced diet is variety. Eating a wide range of foods ensures you get a mix of different nutrients your body needs to function properly. Imagine your diet as a colourful palette—you want to include a variety of fruits, vegetables, grains, proteins, and fats to cover all your nutritional bases.

Fruits and Vegetables:

Aim to fill half your plate with fruits and vegetables. They are rich in vitamins, minerals, fiber, and antioxidants that help protect against chronic diseases.

Whole Grains:

Include whole grains like brown rice, quinoa, and whole-wheat bread, which provide essential nutrients and fiber

.

Proteins:

Incorporate a mix of protein sources, such as lean meats, fish, eggs, beans, nuts, and seeds. Protein is crucial for building and repairing tissues.

Healthy Fats:

Don't shy away from fats, but choose healthy ones like those found in avocados, nuts, seeds, and olive oil. These fats support brain health and hormone production.

Moderation: Finding the Right Balance

Moderation is all about consuming the right amounts of different foods. It's okay to enjoy your favourite treats, but the key is to do so in moderation. Here's how you can practice moderation without feeling deprived:

Portion Control:

Pay attention to serving sizes. Using smaller plates and bowls can help you control portions and avoid overeating.

Mindful Eating:

Focus on your food, savor each bite, and listen to your body's hunger and fullness cues. This can prevent overeating and make meals more satisfying.

Balanced Meals:

Aim for balanced meals that include a mix of macronutrients—carbohydrates, proteins, and fats. This balance helps maintain energy levels and keeps you feeling full longer.

Adequacy: Meeting Nutritional Needs

A balanced diet must provide enough essential nutrients to meet your body's needs. This means getting sufficient vitamins, minerals, proteins, fats, and carbohydrates to support your overall health and well-being.

<u>Micronutrients:</u>

Ensure you're getting enough vitamins and minerals by eating a variety of nutrient-dense foods. For example, leafy greens for iron and calcium, citrus fruits for vitamin C, and dairy or fortified plant milks for vitamin D.

<u>Macronutrients:</u>

Balance your intake of carbohydrates, proteins, and fats. Each macronutrient plays a unique role in your body's function and health.

Proportionality: Balancing Nutrient Intake

Proportionality refers to getting the right balance of nutrients in relation to each other. Different food groups should make up specific proportions of your diet to ensure a balanced intake of nutrients.

<u>Plate Method:</u>

A simple way to visualize proportionality is the plate method. Fill half your plate with vegetables and fruits, a quarter with lean protein, and the remaining quarter with whole grains. Add a serving of healthy fat, like a drizzle of olive oil or a small handful of nuts.

Dietary Guidelines:

Refer to dietary guidelines and recommendations for proportions of different food groups. For example, the Dietary Guidelines for Americans suggest making half your grains whole and varying your protein sources.

Balance: Integrating All Food Groups

Balance means including all food groups in the right proportions over time. It's not about perfection in every meal but about creating an overall pattern of balanced eating.

Daily and Weekly Balance:

Don't stress about each individual meal. Instead, focus on achieving balance over the course of a day or week. This approach makes it easier to enjoy a variety of foods without feeling restricted.

Flexibility:

Be flexible and adapt your diet based on your needs and preferences. Balance can look different for everyone, and it's important to find what works best for you.

Plan Ahead:

Plan your meals and snacks to ensure a variety of nutrients. Preparing a weekly menu can help you stay organized and make healthier choices.

Stay Hydrated:

Don't forget about fluids. Water is essential for hydration and supports all bodily functions. Aim to drink at least 8 cups of water a day, and more if you're active or in a hot climate.

Limit Processed Foods:

Try to limit processed and sugary foods. These often contain empty calories and can disrupt your nutrient balance.

Cook at Home:

Cooking at home allows you to control ingredients and portions, helping you maintain a balanced diet.

Designing a healthy eating plan based on the principles of a balanced diet is about making informed, mindful choices that nourish your body. It's a holistic approach that goes beyond just counting calories or restricting certain foods. By embracing variety, moderation, adequacy, proportionality, and balance, you can create a sustainable and enjoyable way of eating that supports your health and weight management goals.

Portion Control and Mindful Eating

In the hustle and bustle of our daily lives, it's easy to lose track of how much we're eating. Portion sizes have ballooned over the years, and with it, our waistlines. Yet, the solution to overeating isn't about drastic restrictions or complicated diets—it's about portion control and mindful eating. Let's explore these two powerful strategies that can help you design a healthy eating plan that supports your weight management goals.

The Power of Portion Control

Portion control is about understanding and managing the amount of food you eat. It's not about deprivation but about eating the right amounts to nourish your body without overloading it with excess calories. Here's how you can master the art of portion control:

One of the first steps in portion control is understanding serving sizes. What you think is a single serving might actually be two or three servings according to dietary guidelines. For example, a standard serving of cooked pasta is about half a cup, but most restaurant portions are at least double that amount.

Use Measuring Tools:

Invest in a set of measuring cups, spoons, and a kitchen scale. These tools can help you get a realistic idea of what a serving size looks like.

Read Nutrition Labels:

Pay attention to the serving size listed on food labels. This can help you understand how many servings you're consuming.

Tips for Managing Portions

Use Smaller Plates and Bowls:

Our brains are easily fooled by visual cues. Using smaller plates and bowls can make your portions look more substantial, helping you feel satisfied with less food.

<u>Pre-Portion Snacks:</u>

Instead of eating straight from the bag, pre-portion snacks into smaller containers. This prevents mindless munching and helps you keep track of how much you're eating.

<u>Serve Yourself in the Kitchen:</u>

To avoid the temptation of second helpings, serve your meals in the kitchen rather than at the dining table. This makes it less convenient to go back for more.

<u>Be Mindful of Restaurant Portions:</u>

Restaurant portions are often much larger than what you need. Consider sharing a dish, ordering a half portion, or boxing up half your meal to take home.

Embracing Mindful Eating

Mindful eating is about being fully present during your meals. It's the opposite of eating on autopilot. By paying attention to what and how you eat, you can enjoy your food more and tune into your body's hunger and fullness signals.

Eat Slowly:

Take your time to chew thoroughly and savor each bite. Eating slowly gives your brain a chance to register that you're full, which can help prevent overeating.

Eliminate Distractions:

Try to eat without distractions like TV, smartphones, or computers. This allows you to focus on your food and your body's signals.

Listen to Your Body:

Pay attention to your hunger and fullness cues. Eat when you're hungry and stop when you're comfortably full, not stuffed.

Appreciate Your Food:

Take a moment to appreciate the colors, textures, and flavors of your food. This can enhance your eating experience and make meals more satisfying.

Tips for Practising Mindful Eating

Set a Comfortable Eating Environment:

Create a pleasant and calm eating environment. This can make your meals more enjoyable and help you focus on the act of eating.

Pause Between Bites:

Put your fork down between bites to slow down your eating pace. This small pause can make a big difference in how much you eat.

Check In With Yourself:

Before reaching for a second helping, check in with yourself. Are you still hungry, or are you eating out of habit or for emotional reasons?

Engage Your Senses:

Notice the aroma, taste, and texture of your food. Engaging your senses can make you more aware of your eating experience and help you enjoy your food more.

Combining Portion Control and Mindful Eating

When you combine portion control with mindful eating, you create a powerful approach to managing your diet. Here's how these two strategies work together:

Portion Control Sets the Stage:

By managing portions, you set a framework for how much food is appropriate to eat. This helps prevent overeating from the start.

Mindful Eating Enhances the Experience: Mindful eating ensures that you're fully present and engaged with your meal, helping you enjoy it more and listen to your body's needs.

Practical Applications

Let's put these principles into practice with a simple meal. Imagine you're having a balanced dinner of grilled chicken, roasted vegetables, and quinoa.

Portion Control:

Measure out a serving of each component—3 ounces of chicken, 1 cup of vegetables, and 1/2 cup of quinoa. Use a smaller plate to make the portions look satisfying.

Mindful Eating:

Sit at a table without distractions. Take a moment to appreciate the colors and smells of your meal. Eat slowly, savoring each bite, and putting your fork down between bites. Check in with your hunger and fullness cues as you go.

Portion control and mindful eating are not just strategies—they're a journey to a healthier, more balanced relationship with food. By paying attention to how much you eat and truly savoring each meal, you can design an eating plan that supports your health and weight management goals.

Chapter 5: Special Considerations in Diet and Obesity

Childhood Obesity: Causes and Prevention Strategies

Childhood obesity is a growing concern, with rates increasing at an alarming pace globally. It's a complex issue influenced by a mix of genetic, behavioral, and environmental factors. Understanding the causes and implementing prevention strategies is crucial to combat this epidemic and ensure a healthier future for our children. Let's delve into the root causes of childhood obesity and explore practical, effective strategies to prevent it.

Unhealthy Eating Habits

One of the most significant contributors to childhood obesity is poor dietary choices. Many children consume diets high in calories, sugars, and unhealthy fats while lacking essential nutrients.

Processed Foods:

Convenience foods, such as fast food, snacks, and sugary drinks, are often calorie-dense and nutrient-poor.

Portion Sizes:

Over the years, portion sizes have increased, leading to higher calorie intake.

Lack of Fruits and Vegetables:

Many children do not consume enough fruits and vegetables, missing out on vital vitamins, minerals, and fiber.

Sedentary Lifestyle

With the advent of technology, children are spending more time in front of screens and less time being physically active.

Screen Time:

Excessive use of computers, tablets, smartphones, and television leads to a sedentary lifestyle.

Lack of Physical Activity:

Many children do not engage in enough physical activities, such as playing outside, sports, or even simple exercises like walking.

Genetic Factors

Genetics can play a role in childhood obesity. Children with obese parents are more likely to become obese due to inherited traits and learned behaviors.

Family History:

Genetics can influence how a child's body stores and processes fat.

Parental Influence:

Parents' eating habits and activity levels can significantly impact their children's behaviors and weight.

<u>Environmental and Socioeconomic Factors</u>

The environment in which a child grows up can influence their risk of obesity.

<u>Access to Healthy Foods:</u>

Children living in food deserts may have limited access to healthy, affordable foods.

<u>Safe Spaces for Activity:</u>

Lack of safe parks or recreational areas can limit opportunities for physical activity.

<u>Socioeconomic Status:</u>

Families with limited financial resources might rely more on cheap, high-calorie foods and have less access to health education.

Prevention Strategies for Childhood Obesity

<u>Promote Healthy Eating Habits</u>

Teaching children about nutrition and encouraging healthy eating habits from a young age can make a significant difference.

Balanced Meals:

Ensure meals include a variety of fruits, vegetables, whole grains, lean proteins, and healthy fats.

Limit Sugary Drinks and Snacks:

Reduce the consumption of sugary beverages and unhealthy snacks. Encourage water and healthy snacks like fruits and nuts.

Family Meals:

Eating together as a family can model healthy eating habits and provide opportunities for parents to teach children about balanced diets.

Encourage Physical Activity

Incorporating physical activity into daily routines can help children maintain a healthy weight and develop a love for movement.

Active Play:

Encourage children to play outside, engage in sports, or participate in physical activities they enjoy.

Limit Screen Time:

Set limits on screen time and promote other activities like reading, hobbies, or family outings.

Family Activities:

Plan active family outings, such as hiking, biking, or playing games in the park, to make exercise a fun and regular part of life.

Educate and Empower

Providing education and resources to both children and parents can empower them to make healthier choices.

School Programs:

Support school programs that educate children about nutrition and the importance of physical activity.

Health Education:

Provide parents with information and resources to help them make healthier food choices and create an active lifestyle for the whole family.

Community Resources:

Utilize community programs and resources, such as local fitness centers, farmers' markets, and health workshops.

<u>Create Supportive Environments</u>

Creating environments that support healthy lifestyles is essential for long-term success in preventing childhood obesity.

<u>Healthy School Environments:</u>

Advocate for healthier school meals and opportunities for physical activity during the school day.

<u>Community Initiatives:</u>

Support community initiatives that improve access to healthy foods and safe places for physical activity.

<u>Policy Changes:</u>

Encourage policies that promote health, such as limiting the marketing of unhealthy foods to children and improving food labeling.

<u>Conclusion: Building a Healthier Future</u>

Addressing childhood obesity requires a comprehensive approach that includes healthy eating, physical activity, education, and supportive environments. By understanding the causes and implementing effective prevention strategies, we can help children achieve and maintain a healthy weight, setting the foundation for a healthier future.

Pregnancy and Obesity: Dietary Recommendations

Pregnancy is a transformative journey filled with excitement, anticipation, and countless questions about how to ensure the best outcomes for both mother and baby. For women dealing with obesity, pregnancy brings additional considerations and challenges. Proper nutrition is paramount, not only for the health of the baby but also for the well-being of the mother. Let's explore the unique dietary needs during pregnancy for women with obesity and how thoughtful dietary choices can make a significant difference.

The Impact of Obesity on Pregnancy

Obesity during pregnancy can increase the risk of complications such as gestational diabetes, preeclampsia, and cesarean delivery. It can also affect the baby's health, potentially leading to higher birth weight and an increased risk of obesity later in life. However, with the right dietary recommendations, these risks can be managed and minimized.

The Goals of a Healthy Pregnancy Diet

The primary goals for a healthy pregnancy diet for women with obesity include:

Supporting Fetal Development:

Ensuring the baby gets the essential nutrients for proper growth and development.

Maintaining Healthy Weight Gain:

Managing weight gain to avoid excessive increases while still supporting a healthy pregnancy.

Preventing Complications:

Reducing the risk of gestational diabetes, hypertension, and other obesity-related complications.

Key Dietary Recommendations

Focus on Nutrient-Dense Foods

Nutrient-dense foods provide essential vitamins, minerals, and other nutrients without excessive calories. They are the cornerstone of a healthy pregnancy diet.

<u>Fruits and Vegetables:</u>

Aim for a variety of colours and types to get a wide range of nutrients. Leafy greens, berries, and cruciferous vegetables are particularly beneficial.

<u>Whole Grains:</u>

Opt for whole grains like quinoa, brown rice, and whole-wheat bread instead of refined grains.

<u>Lean Proteins:</u>

Include lean protein sources such as chicken, turkey, fish, beans, and legumes. These help support fetal growth and maternal health.

<u>Healthy Fats:</u>

Incorporate healthy fats from sources like avocados, nuts, seeds, and olive oil. These fats are crucial for fetal brain development.

<u>Manage Caloric Intake</u>

While it's important to nourish both mother and baby, managing caloric intake helps prevent excessive weight gain.

Caloric Needs:

Consult with a healthcare provider to determine the appropriate caloric intake based on individual needs and stage of pregnancy.

Mindful Eating:

Practice mindful eating by paying attention to hunger and fullness cues. Avoid eating out of boredom or stress.

Small, Frequent Meals:

Eating small, frequent meals can help manage hunger and maintain energy levels throughout the day.

Monitor Carbohydrate Intake

Carbohydrates are a vital energy source but need to be managed carefully, especially to prevent gestational diabetes.

Choose Complex Carbohydrates:

Opt for complex carbohydrates such as whole grains, legumes, and vegetables. These provide sustained energy and important nutrients.

Limit Simple Carbohydrates:

Reduce intake of simple carbohydrates found in sugary snacks, desserts, and refined grains.

Stay Hydrated

Proper hydration supports overall health and can help manage pregnancy-related symptoms such as swelling and constipation.

Water Intake:

Aim for at least 8-10 glasses of water per day, more if you're active or live in a hot climate.

Avoid Sugary Drinks:

Limit or avoid sugary drinks like soda and fruit juices. Opt for water, herbal teas, or infused water with fruits for flavour.

Special Considerations

Prenatal Vitamins

Prenatal vitamins are essential to fill any nutritional gaps and ensure the baby gets the necessary nutrients.

Folic Acid:

Essential for preventing neural tube defects. Aim for at least 400-800 micrograms per day.

Iron:

Supports the increased blood volume during pregnancy. Include iron-rich foods and consider an iron supplement if recommended by a healthcare provider.

Calcium and Vitamin D:

Important for bone health. Include dairy or fortified plant-based alternatives, and consider supplements if needed.

Monitoring Weight Gain

Weight gain during pregnancy should be monitored carefully. The recommended weight gain varies based on pre-pregnancy BMI.

Guidelines:

For women with obesity, the recommended weight gain during pregnancy is typically lower than for women with a normal BMI. Consult with a healthcare provider for personalized recommendations.

Regular Check-Ins:

Regular prenatal visits help monitor weight gain and adjust dietary plans as needed.

Addressing Gestational Diabetes

Women with obesity are at higher risk for gestational diabetes, which requires careful management.

Blood Sugar Monitoring:

Regularly monitor blood sugar levels as advised by a healthcare provider.

Dietary Adjustments:

Focus on a balanced diet with controlled carbohydrate intake to manage blood sugar levels.

Physical Activity:

Engage in safe, moderate physical activity as approved by a healthcare provider to help regulate blood sugar.

Practical Tips for a Healthy Pregnancy Diet

Meal Planning:

Plan meals ahead of time to ensure a balanced diet and avoid last-minute unhealthy choices.

<u>Healthy Snacking:</u>

Keep healthy snacks on hand, such as nuts, yogurt, fruits, and vegetable sticks, to manage hunger between meals.

<u>Cooking at Home:</u>

Prepare meals at home to control ingredients and portions, making it easier to stick to dietary recommendations.

<u>Seek Support:</u>

Don't hesitate to seek support from healthcare providers, dietitians, or support groups to help navigate dietary changes during pregnancy.

Pregnancy is a critical time for both mother and baby, and proper nutrition plays a vital role in ensuring a healthy outcome. For women with obesity, thoughtful dietary recommendations can help manage risks and support a healthy, successful pregnancy. By focusing on nutrient-dense foods, managing caloric intake, and addressing special considerations, you can create a nurturing environment that promotes health for both you and your baby.

Obesity and Diabetes

Obesity and diabetes are two interlinked conditions that have reached epidemic proportions worldwide. Their relationship is complex, yet understanding it is crucial for managing and preventing both. This section explores the intricate connection between obesity and diabetes, delves into the science behind it, and offers practical dietary strategies to manage and mitigate the risks.

The Obesity-Diabetes Connection

Obesity, particularly excess abdominal fat, significantly increases the risk of developing type 2 diabetes. Here's why:

Insulin Resistance

Obesity often leads to insulin resistance, a condition where the body's cells become less responsive to insulin. Insulin is a hormone that helps glucose enter cells to be used as energy. When cells resist insulin, glucose accumulates in the bloodstream, leading to elevated blood sugar levels and eventually type 2 diabetes.

Inflammation

Excess fat tissue, especially around the abdomen, releases inflammatory substances known as adipokines. Chronic inflammation can disrupt the function of insulin and further exacerbate insulin resistance.

Beta-Cell Dysfunction

The pancreas has to work harder to produce more insulin to overcome insulin resistance. Over time, the insulin-producing beta cells in the pancreas can become dysfunctional and less effective, contributing to the progression of type 2 diabetes.

The Role of Diet in Managing Obesity and Diabetes

Diet plays a pivotal role in managing both obesity and diabetes. By making informed dietary choices, individuals can improve insulin sensitivity, control blood sugar levels, and achieve a healthy weight. Here are some key dietary strategies:

Embrace a Balanced Diet

A balanced diet that includes a variety of nutrients is essential for overall health and managing diabetes.

Complex Carbohydrates:

Opt for complex carbohydrates such as whole grains, legumes, and vegetables. These have a lower glycemic index (GI), meaning they release glucose more slowly into the bloodstream.

<u>Lean Proteins:</u>

Include lean protein sources like poultry, fish, beans, and low-fat dairy. Proteins help stabilize blood sugar levels and promote satiety.

<u>Healthy Fats:</u>

Incorporate healthy fats from sources like avocados, nuts, seeds, and olive oil. These fats can improve insulin sensitivity and support heart health.

<u>Fruits and Vegetables:</u>

Aim for a colourful variety of fruits and vegetables to ensure adequate intake of vitamins, minerals, and fiber.

<u>Monitor Carbohydrate Intake</u>

Carbohydrates have the most direct impact on blood sugar levels. Managing carbohydrate intake is crucial for individuals with diabetes.

Carb Counting:

Learn to count carbohydrates to help manage blood sugar levels. Work with a dietitian to determine the appropriate amount of carbs per meal.

Portion Control:

Be mindful of portion sizes to avoid consuming excess carbohydrates that can spike blood sugar levels.

Focus on Fiber

Fiber slows down the digestion and absorption of carbohydrates, leading to a more gradual rise in blood sugar levels.

Whole Foods:

Choose whole foods rich in fiber, such as vegetables, fruits, whole grains, and legumes.

Daily Goal:

Aim for at least 25-30 grams of fiber per day.

Limit Added Sugars

Added sugars can cause rapid spikes in blood sugar levels and contribute to weight gain.

Read Labels:

Check food labels for added sugars, which are often hidden in processed foods and beverages.

Natural Sweeteners:

Consider natural sweeteners like stevia or monk fruit as alternatives to sugar.

Stay Hydrated

Proper hydration is important for overall health and can help manage blood sugar levels.

Water:

Water should be the primary beverage of choice.

Avoid Sugary Drinks:

Limit sugary drinks like sodas, energy drinks, and sweetened teas, which can cause blood sugar spikes.

Managing obesity and diabetes through diet is a journey that requires knowledge, commitment, and support. By understanding the connection between obesity and diabetes and implementing effective dietary strategies, individuals can take control of their health and improve their quality of life.

Chapter 6: Psychological Aspects of Eating

Emotional Eating and Stress Management

Imagine this: you've had a stressful day at work, you drive home feeling tired and drained and the moment you walk through your door, you find yourself reaching for that tub of ice cream in the freezer or the bag of chips in the kitchen cupboards. It's not hunger driving you; it's a need for comfort, a way to soothe the emotional storm within. This is emotional eating, a common response to stress and a significant factor in the struggle with obesity. Let's explore the relationship between emotional eating and stress, and discover strategies to manage them effectively.

The Comfort of Food

Food often serves as a coping mechanism for dealing with emotions. When stressed, anxious, or sad, turning to food can provide a temporary sense of relief and comfort.

Comfort Foods:

Typically, comfort foods are high in sugar, fat, and carbohydrates, which can trigger the brain's reward system and release feel-good chemicals like dopamine.

Emotional Triggers:

Common emotional triggers for eating include stress, boredom, loneliness, anger, and fatigue.

The Biological Response

Stress affects the body's biology, influencing eating behaviors in several ways.

Cortisol:

When stressed, the body releases cortisol, a hormone that can increase appetite and cravings for high-calorie foods.

Insulin Resistance:

Chronic stress can lead to insulin resistance, which can further increase hunger and cravings.

Identifying Emotional Eating Patterns

The first step in managing emotional eating is to recognize when it happens and understand the triggers.

Mindful Awareness

Becoming aware of your eating patterns and the emotions driving them is crucial.

Food Diary:

Keep a food diary to track what you eat, when you eat, and what emotions you're experiencing at the time. This can help identify patterns and triggers.

Mindfulness:

Practice mindfulness to stay present and aware of your thoughts and feelings. This can help differentiate between physical hunger and emotional hunger.

Understanding Triggers

Identify the specific emotions or situations that trigger emotional eating.

<u>Stressful Events:</u>

Notice if stressful events at work, school, or home lead to cravings for certain foods.

<u>Emotional States:</u>

Pay attention to whether feelings of sadness, loneliness, or boredom prompt you to eat.

Strategies for Managing Emotional Eating

Once you've identified the triggers and patterns, the next step is to develop strategies to manage emotional eating and reduce stress.

<u>Healthy Coping Mechanisms</u>

Find alternative ways to cope with emotions that don't involve food.

<u>Exercise:</u>

Physical activity can reduce stress, improve mood, and serve as a healthy outlet for emotions. Even a short walk can make a difference.

Relaxation Techniques:

Practices like deep breathing, meditation, and yoga can help calm the mind and body.

Hobbies:

Engage in hobbies and activities you enjoy, such as reading, painting, or gardening, to divert your focus from food.

Balanced Nutrition

Adopt a balanced diet to maintain steady blood sugar levels and reduce cravings.

Regular Meals:

Eat regular, balanced meals to prevent extreme hunger, which can trigger emotional eating.

Nutrient-Dense Foods:

Focus on nutrient-dense foods that provide sustained energy and satisfy hunger, such as whole grains, lean proteins, fruits, and vegetables.

Healthy Snacks:

Keep healthy snacks on hand, such as nuts, yogurt, or fruit, to avoid reaching for junk food when emotions strike.

Stress Management Techniques

Effective stress management can reduce the urge to turn to food for comfort.

Time Management:

Improve your time management skills to reduce stress from deadlines and busy schedules.

Social Support:

Build a support network of friends, family, or support groups to share your feelings and experiences.

Professional Help:

Consider seeking help from a therapist or counsellor to address underlying emotional issues and develop healthy coping strategies.

Practical Tips for Everyday Life

Incorporating these strategies into daily life can help you manage emotional eating and stress more effectively.

Plan Ahead

Planning your meals and snacks can help you make healthier choices even when emotions run high.

Meal Prep:

Prepare healthy meals and snacks in advance to have readily available options.

Shopping List:

Make a shopping list and stick to it to avoid buying impulsive, unhealthy foods.

Create a Supportive Environment

Set up your environment to support healthier eating habits and stress management.

Healthy Environment:

Keep your home stocked with healthy foods and limit the availability of high-calorie, comfort foods.

Stress-Free Zones:

Designate areas in your home for relaxation and stress-relief activities, such as a cozy reading nook or a yoga corner.

Practice Self-Compassion

Be kind to yourself and recognize that it's okay to have setbacks.

<u>Forgive Yourself:</u>
If you slip into emotional eating, forgive yourself and focus on making healthier choices going forward.

<u>Positive Affirmations:</u>
Use positive affirmations to reinforce your commitment to healthy eating and stress management.

Emotional eating is a common challenge, but with awareness and practical strategies, it's possible to break the cycle and achieve a healthier relationship with food. By managing stress and developing healthier coping mechanisms, you can nurture both your emotional and physical well-being.

Strategies for Behavior Change and Sustaining Healthy Habits

When it comes to diet and obesity, it's clear that the physical aspects of what we eat are only part of the picture. Our eating behaviors, shaped by habits, emotions, and psychological factors, play a significant role. Changing these behaviors and maintaining healthy habits can be challenging, but it's crucial for long-term success. In this section, we'll explore effective strategies for behavior change and how to sustain these healthy habits over time.

Understanding Behavior Change

Behaviour change is a process that involves several stages. Recognizing where you are in this process can help tailor your approach to making lasting changes.

The Stages of Change Model

Developed by psychologists James Prochaska and Carlo DiClemente, the Stages of Change Model outlines five key stages people typically go through when modifying behaviour:

Precontemplation:

Not yet considering change.

Contemplation:

Acknowledging the need for change but not ready to start.

Preparation:

Getting ready to change.

<u>Action:</u>

Actively working on changing behaviour

.

<u>Maintenance:</u>

Sustaining the new behaviour over time.

Understanding which stage you're in can help you apply the right strategies to move forward.

Strategies for Behavior Change

<u>Set SMART Goals</u>

Setting goals is a fundamental part of behaviour change, but it's essential that these goals are SMART:

<u>Specific:</u>

Clearly define what you want to achieve.

<u>Measurable:</u>

Ensure you can track your progress.

<u>Achievable:</u>

Set realistic and attainable goals.

<u>Relevant:</u>

Make sure your goals align with your overall objectives.

<u>Time-bound:</u>

Set a deadline to create a sense of urgency.

For example, instead of saying, "I want to eat healthier," you could set a SMART goal like, "I will eat at least five servings of fruits and vegetables every day for the next month."

Identify Triggers and Cues

Understanding what triggers unhealthy eating behaviours can help you develop strategies to avoid or manage these situations.

Environmental Triggers:

Identify and modify your environment to reduce exposure to unhealthy food cues, such as keeping junk food out of the house.

Emotional Triggers:

Recognize emotional states that lead to unhealthy eating, such as stress or boredom, and develop alternative coping mechanisms.

Develop Healthy Routines

Routines and habits form the backbone of behaviour change. Creating new, healthier routines can help replace old, unhealthy habits.

Consistent Meal Times:

Establish regular meal times to avoid random snacking and ensure balanced nutrition throughout the day.

Healthy Snacking:

Keep healthy snacks on hand, such as fruits, nuts, or yogurt, to avoid reaching for less nutritious options.

Use Positive Reinforcement

Positive reinforcement involves rewarding yourself for making healthy choices, which can help reinforce these behaviours.

Non-Food Rewards:

Choose rewards that don't involve food, such as a new book, a massage, or a fun outing.

Celebrate Small Wins:

Recognize and celebrate small milestones along the way to stay motivated.

Sustaining Healthy Habits

Once you've made changes, sustaining these healthy habits is crucial for long-term success. Here are some strategies to help maintain your progress:

Build a Support System

Having a support system can make a significant difference in maintaining healthy habits.

Family and Friends:

Involve family and friends in your journey. Their support can provide encouragement and accountability.

Support Groups:

Join a support group or community with similar goals. Sharing experiences and tips can help keep you motivated.

Monitor Your Progress

Regularly tracking your progress can help you stay on course and make adjustments as needed.

Journaling:

Keep a food and activity journal to monitor your habits and identify areas for improvement.

Apps and Tools:

Use apps or digital tools to track your food intake, exercise, and progress towards your goals.

Stay Flexible and Adaptable

Life is full of changes and challenges, and flexibility is key to sustaining healthy habits.

Adjust Goals:

Be willing to adjust your goals and strategies as needed based on your progress and any new challenges that arise.

Learn from Setbacks:

View setbacks as learning opportunities rather than failures. Analyze what went wrong and develop a plan to overcome similar obstacles in the future.

Practice Mindfulness

Mindfulness can help you stay present and aware of your eating habits and overall well-being.

Mindful Eating:

Practice mindful eating by paying attention to your hunger and fullness cues, savoring each bite, and avoiding distractions during meals.

Stress Management:

Incorporate mindfulness techniques like meditation, deep breathing, or yoga to manage stress and prevent emotional eating.

Practical Tips for Sustaining Healthy Habits

Plan and Prepare

Planning and preparation can help you stay on track with your healthy habits.

Meal Prep:

Prepare meals in advance to ensure you have healthy options readily available.

Grocery Shopping:

Make a shopping list based on your meal plan and stick to it to avoid impulse buys.

Make it Enjoyable

Find ways to make healthy eating and exercise enjoyable and satisfying.

Experiment with Recipes:

Try new recipes and cooking methods to keep meals exciting and varied.

Find Fun Activities:

Choose physical activities you enjoy, whether it's dancing, hiking, or playing a sport.

By setting realistic goals, identifying triggers, developing routines, and building a support system, you can create lasting changes that support your health and well-being.

Chapter 7: Practical Tips for Grocery Shopping and Meal Preparation

Reading Food Labels: Understanding Nutrient Content

Picture this: you're standing in the grocery aisle, faced with a myriad of choices. Colorful packaging, bold health claims, and an overwhelming array of options can make it difficult to know what's actually good for you. This is where understanding how to read food labels comes into play. Mastering this skill can transform your shopping experience and help you make informed, healthier choices. Let's dive into the art of decoding food labels and understanding nutrient content.

The Importance of Food Labels

Food labels are a treasure trove of information, offering insights into what you're really putting into your body. They can help you:

Make healthier choices:

Identify products that fit your dietary needs.

Manage portion sizes:

Understand serving sizes to avoid overeating.

Spot hidden ingredients:

Avoid unwanted additives and allergens.

Breaking Down the Food Label

A typical food label contains several key sections. Here's a guide to what each part means and how to interpret it:

Serving Size

At the top of the label, you'll find the serving size and the number of servings per container. This is crucial because all the nutritional information provided is based on this serving size.

<u>Tip:</u>

Compare the serving size to how much you actually eat. If you're consuming more or less than the serving size, adjust the nutritional information accordingly.

<u>Calories</u>

The calorie section tells you how many calories are in one serving of the product. This is important for managing your overall energy intake.

<u>Tip:</u>

Keep in mind your daily calorie needs, which can vary based on age, sex, and activity level.

<u>Nutrients to Limit</u>

Look next at the nutrients you might want to limit in your diet, such as saturated fat, trans fat, cholesterol, and sodium. Excessive intake of these can lead to health issues like heart disease and high blood pressure.

<u>Saturated and Trans Fats:</u>

These can raise LDL (bad) cholesterol levels. Aim to minimize their intake.

<u>Cholesterol:</u>

High intake can also affect heart health. Try to keep it in check.

<u>Sodium:</u>

Too much sodium can increase blood pressure. Look for lower-sodium options.

<u>Nutrients to Get More Of</u>

Focus on the beneficial nutrients that you need more of in your diet, such as dietary fiber, vitamins (like A and C), calcium, and iron.

<u>Dietary Fiber:</u>

Helps with digestion and can keep you feeling full longer.

<u>Vitamins and Minerals:</u>

Essential for various body functions and overall health. Check for products rich in these nutrients.

<u>% Daily Value (%DV)</u>

The %DV indicates how much of a nutrient one serving of the food contributes to a daily diet, based on a 2,000-calorie diet.

<u>Low vs. High:</u>

5% DV or less of a nutrient is considered low, while 20% DV or more is high. Use this to gauge if a food is high or low in specific nutrients.

<u>Decoding Ingredients Lists</u>

The ingredients list provides a detailed look at what's in your food. Ingredients are listed in descending order by weight.

<u>First Ingredients:</u>

Pay attention to the first few ingredients, as they make up the bulk of the product. If sugar, fat, or salt is listed first, the product might not be the healthiest choice.

<u>Hidden Sugars:</u>

Sugar can appear under many names like high fructose corn syrup, cane sugar, or agave nectar. Be aware of these aliases.

<u>Whole Foods:</u>

Look for products with whole food ingredients like whole grains, vegetables, and lean proteins.

Practical Tips for Reading Labels

Now that you understand the components of a food label, here are some practical tips to make label reading easier:

Compare Products

Use food labels to compare similar products. Choose the option with the better nutrient profile.

Example:

When choosing between two cereals, compare their fiber, sugar, and sodium content.

Be Skeptical of Marketing Claims

Health claims on the front of packaging can be misleading. Always verify these claims by checking the actual nutritional information on the back.

Example:

A product labeled "low fat" might be high in sugar to compensate for taste.

Don't Forget Serving Sizes

Always factor in the serving size. A small-looking package might contain multiple servings, meaning you could be consuming more calories and nutrients than intended.

<u>Look for Whole Grains</u>

For bread, pasta, and cereals, look for whole grains listed as the first ingredient. Whole grains are more nutritious and provide more fiber than refined grains.

Reading food labels is an essential skill for anyone looking to maintain a healthy diet and manage their weight. It empowers you to make informed decisions, avoid unhealthy ingredients, and choose foods that support your health goals. By taking a few moments to understand the labels, you're taking a big step towards a healthier, more informed way of eating.

Healthy Cooking Techniques and Recipes

Cooking at home is one of the most empowering ways to take control of your diet and health. But healthy cooking doesn't have to be bland or boring. With the right techniques and recipes, you can prepare delicious meals that are both nutritious and satisfying. Let's explore some healthy cooking methods and share a few recipes to get you started on your culinary adventure.

Healthy Cooking Techniques

Adopting healthy cooking techniques is key to reducing unhealthy fats, added sugars, and excess calories in your meals. Here are some methods to keep in mind:

Steaming

Steaming is a great way to cook vegetables, fish, and poultry without adding extra fat. It helps retain the nutrients and natural flavors of the food.

How to Steam:

Use a steamer basket over boiling water or an electric steamer. Season with herbs and spices for added flavor.

Grilling

Grilling adds a smoky flavor to foods while allowing excess fat to drip away, making it a healthier option for cooking meats and vegetables.

How to Grill:

Preheat the grill, lightly oil the grates, and cook foods over direct or indirect heat. Use marinades to enhance the taste.

Baking and Roasting

Baking and roasting use dry heat to cook foods evenly, preserving their natural flavors and textures. This method works well for vegetables, lean meats, and whole grains.

How to Bake/Roast:

Preheat the oven, arrange food on a baking sheet, and cook at the recommended temperature. Use parchment paper or silicone mats to reduce the need for added fats.

Sautéing and Stir-Frying

These quick-cooking methods use a small amount of healthy oil and high heat to cook food rapidly, preserving nutrients and flavors.

How to Sauté/Stir-Fry:

Heat a small amount of oil (such as olive or avocado oil) in a pan, add your ingredients, and cook while stirring frequently.

Poaching

Poaching involves cooking food gently in simmering liquid, which can help retain moisture and reduce the need for added fats.

<u>How to Poach:</u>

Use water, broth, or wine to gently cook proteins like fish, chicken, or eggs. Keep the liquid just below boiling.

Delicious and Healthy Recipes

Here are some simple, healthy recipes to try at home. These dishes are designed to be flavorful, nutritious, and easy to prepare.

<u>Grilled Lemon Herb Chicken</u>

<u>Ingredients:</u>

- 4 boneless, skinless chicken breasts
- 2 tablespoons olive oil
- Juice of 1 lemon
- 2 garlic cloves, minced
- 1 tablespoon fresh thyme leaves
- 1 tablespoon fresh rosemary leaves
- Salt and pepper to taste

<u>Instructions:</u>

1. In a small bowl, mix olive oil, lemon juice,   garlic, thyme, rosemary, salt, and pepper.

2. Place chicken breasts in a resealable plastic bag and pour the marinade over them. Seal the bag and refrigerate for at least 30 minutes.

3. Preheat the grill to medium-high heat.

4. Remove chicken from the marinade and grill for 6-7 minutes on each side, or until cooked through.

5. Serve with a side of steamed vegetables or a fresh salad.

<u>Quinoa and Vegetable Stir-Fry</u>

Ingredients:

- 1 cup quinoa, rinsed

- 2 cups water or vegetable broth

- 1 tablespoon olive oil

- 1 red bell pepper, sliced

- 1 yellow bell pepper, sliced

- 1 cup snap peas

- 1 carrot, julienned

- 2 garlic cloves, minced

- 1 tablespoon soy sauce (low sodium)

- 1 tablespoon sesame oil

- 1 tablespoon fresh ginger, grated

- 2 green onions, sliced

Instructions:

1. In a medium pot, bring quinoa and water or broth to a boil. Reduce heat, cover, and simmer for 15 minutes, or until quinoa is tender and water is absorbed.

2. In a large skillet, heat olive oil over medium-high heat. Add bell peppers, snap peas, carrot, and garlic. Sauté for 5-7 minutes.

3. Add cooked quinoa to the skillet along with soy sauce, sesame oil, and ginger. Stir to combine and cook for another 2-3 minutes.

4. Garnish with green onions and serve.

<u>Baked Salmon with Asparagus</u>

Ingredients:

- 4 salmon fillets

- 1 bunch asparagus, trimmed

- 2 tablespoons olive oil

- Juice of 1 lemon

- 2 garlic cloves, minced

- Salt and pepper to taste

- Fresh dill or parsley for garnish

Instructions:

1. Preheat the oven to 400°F (200°C).

2. Place salmon fillets and asparagus on a baking sheet lined with parchment paper.

3. Drizzle olive oil and lemon juice over the salmon and asparagus. Sprinkle with garlic, salt, and pepper.

4. Bake for 15-20 minutes, or until salmon is cooked through and asparagus is tender.

5. Garnish with fresh dill or parsley and serve with a side of quinoa or brown rice.

Plan Your Meals

Planning your meals ahead of time can help you make healthier choices and save time during the week.

Meal Prep:

Set aside time each week to plan and prepare meals. Cook in batches and store portions in the fridge or freezer.

Grocery List:

Make a grocery list based on your meal plan to ensure you have all the necessary ingredients.

Use Fresh Ingredients

Fresh, whole ingredients are the foundation of healthy meals. Aim to incorporate a variety of fruits, vegetables, whole grains, lean proteins, and healthy fats.

Reduce Added Sugars and Salt

Be mindful of added sugars and salt in your cooking. Use herbs, spices, and natural flavors to enhance the taste of your dishes.

Natural Sweeteners:

Use honey, maple syrup, or fruit to sweeten dishes naturally.

Herbs and Spices:

Experiment with different herbs and spices to add flavor without extra sodium.

Healthy cooking techniques and nutritious recipes are key components of a balanced diet and a healthier lifestyle. By mastering these skills, you can enjoy delicious meals that support your health goals and make eating well a pleasurable experience. Remember, cooking at home gives you control over the ingredients and preparation methods, allowing you to make choices that benefit your body and well-being.

Chapter 8: Physical Activity and its Role in Weight Management

Combining Diet with Exercise: Synergistic Effects

When it comes to weight management, the combination of a balanced diet and regular exercise is the ultimate power duo. While each can be effective on its own, together they create a synergistic effect that amplifies your results, helping you achieve and maintain a healthy weight more efficiently. Let's explore how diet and exercise work together to support your weight management goals and overall well-being.

The Dynamic Duo: Diet and Exercise

Think of your body as a high-performance machine. To operate optimally, it needs the right fuel (diet) and regular maintenance (exercise). Here's how these two elements complement each other:

Boosting Metabolism

Diet and exercise both play crucial roles in regulating your metabolism—the process by which your body converts food into energy. A nutritious diet provides the essential nutrients your body needs, while exercise increases your metabolic rate, helping you burn more calories even at rest.

Diet:

Eating a diet rich in whole foods, lean proteins, healthy fats, and complex carbohydrates can keep your metabolism running smoothly.

Exercise:

Regular physical activity, especially strength training, builds muscle mass, which burns more calories than fat tissue, boosting your basal metabolic rate (BMR).

Enhancing Weight Loss

Combining diet with exercise helps create a calorie deficit, which is necessary for weight loss. By consuming fewer calories than you burn, your body starts to use stored fat for energy, leading to weight loss.

<u>Diet:</u>

Reducing calorie intake through portion control and healthier food choices is essential for creating a calorie deficit.

<u>Exercise:</u>

Physical activity helps increase the number of calories you burn, making it easier to achieve and maintain a calorie deficit.

<u>Improving Body Composition</u>

While losing weight is a common goal, improving body composition—reducing fat while preserving or building muscle—is often more important for long-term health and aesthetics. Diet and exercise work together to achieve this balance.

<u>Diet:</u>

Consuming adequate protein supports muscle repair and growth, especially after exercise.

<u>Exercise:</u>

Strength training and cardiovascular exercises help build and maintain muscle mass while reducing body fat.

The Synergistic Effect

When diet and exercise are combined, their benefits extend beyond weight management. Here's a look at some of the synergistic effects:

Better Blood Sugar Control

A balanced diet and regular exercise can improve insulin sensitivity, helping your body regulate blood sugar levels more effectively.

Diet:

Eating complex carbohydrates, fiber, and healthy fats helps stabilize blood sugar levels.

Exercise:

Physical activity enhances your muscles' ability to absorb glucose, reducing the risk of insulin resistance and type 2 diabetes.

Enhanced Mental Health

The combination of a healthy diet and exercise has profound effects on mental well-being.

<u>Diet:</u>

Nutrient-rich foods support brain health and can improve mood and cognitive function.

<u>Exercise:</u>

Physical activity releases endorphins, the body's natural mood lifters, and can reduce symptoms of depression and anxiety.

<u>Increased Energy Levels</u>

A nutritious diet fuels your body, while exercise improves circulation and cardiovascular health, leading to higher energy levels and reduced fatigue.

<u>Diet:</u>

Consuming a variety of nutrient-dense foods ensures your body gets the vitamins and minerals it needs for sustained energy.

<u>Exercise:</u>

Regular physical activity increases stamina and reduces feelings of tiredness over time.

To harness the synergistic effects of diet and exercise, consider these practical tips:

Set Realistic Goals

Establish achievable goals for both diet and exercise. Whether it's losing a certain amount of weight, running a 5K, or simply eating more vegetables, clear objectives can keep you motivated.

Plan Your Meals and Workouts

Create a weekly meal plan and workout schedule. Planning helps ensure you're eating balanced meals and making time for regular physical activity.

Meal Prep:

Prepare healthy meals and snacks in advance to avoid the temptation of unhealthy options.

Workout Routine:

Schedule workouts at a convenient time and treat them like important appointments.

Pay attention to how your body responds to different foods and exercises. Adjust your diet and workout regimen based on your energy levels, performance, and recovery.

Hydration:

Stay hydrated, especially before, during, and after exercise.

Recovery:

Allow time for rest and recovery to prevent overtraining and injury.

Sample Synergistic Routine

Here's a simple routine to help you combine diet and exercise effectively:

Morning

Breakfast:

A balanced meal with protein, healthy fats, and complex carbs (e.g., Greek yogurt with nuts and berries).

Workout:

A 30-minute cardio session (e.g., jogging, cycling, or a HIIT workout).

Midday:

<u>Lunch:</u>

A nutrient-dense salad with lean protein, plenty of vegetables, and a healthy fat source (e.g., grilled chicken salad with avocado).

<u>Afternoon</u>

<u>Snack:</u>

A piece of fruit or a handful of nuts to keep energy levels steady.

<u>Evening</u>

<u>Dinner:</u>

A well-balanced meal with protein, whole grains, and vegetables (e.g., baked salmon, quinoa, and steamed broccoli).

<u>Workout:</u>

A 30-minute strength training session or yoga for flexibility and relaxation.

Combining diet and exercise is not just about losing weight; it's about creating a sustainable lifestyle that promotes overall health and well-being. By understanding how these elements work together and implementing practical strategies, you can harness their synergistic power to achieve your health goals. Remember, the journey to a healthier you is a marathon, not a sprint. Consistency and balance are key.

Types of Physical Activities for Different Fitness Levels

When it comes to incorporating physical activity into your weight management plan, it's essential to choose exercises that match your fitness level. Whether you're just starting out or are already a seasoned athlete, there's a type of physical activity that's perfect for you. Let's explore various exercises suited for different fitness levels to help you find the right fit for your lifestyle and goals.

For Beginners: Building the Foundation

Starting your fitness journey can be both exciting and intimidating, but the key is to ease into it. Focus on low-impact, accessible activities that gradually build your strength and endurance.

<u>Walking</u>

Walking is one of the simplest and most effective forms of exercise. It's easy on the joints, requires no special equipment, and can be done anywhere.

<u>Why it works:</u>

Walking helps improve cardiovascular health, burns calories, and boosts mood.

<u>How to start:</u>

Aim for at least 30 minutes a day, whether it's a brisk walk around your neighborhood or a stroll during lunch breaks.

Swimming

Swimming is a full-body workout that's gentle on the joints, making it ideal for beginners or those with joint issues.

<u>Why it works:</u>

It enhances cardiovascular fitness, strengthens muscles, and increases flexibility.

<u>How to start:</u>

Begin with 15-20 minutes of swimming, gradually increasing the duration as your stamina improves.

Yoga

Yoga combines physical postures, breathing exercises, and meditation. It's great for beginners looking to improve flexibility, balance, and stress management.

Why it works:

Yoga promotes relaxation, builds muscle strength, and improves overall flexibility.

How to start:

Join a beginner's yoga class or follow online tutorials. Start with basic poses and gradually progress to more challenging ones.

For Intermediate: Stepping Up the Game

If you've been exercising regularly and are looking to challenge yourself further, intermediate activities can help you build on your existing fitness foundation.

Running

For those who've mastered walking, running is a natural next step. It's an excellent way to boost cardiovascular health and burn calories quickly.

Why it works:

Running enhances heart health, strengthens leg muscles, and can be a great stress reliever.

How to start:

Begin with a mix of walking and running intervals, gradually increasing the running duration as your endurance improves.

Cycling

Cycling is a fantastic cardiovascular workout that also strengthens the lower body. It's great for those looking to increase their intensity while keeping things enjoyable.

Why it works:

Cycling improves heart health, tones leg muscles, and is a low-impact exercise that's easy on the joints.

How to start:

Start with 20-30 minute sessions on a stationary bike or ride outdoors. Gradually increase the distance and intensity.

Pilates

Pilates focuses on core strength, flexibility, and overall body conditioning. It's perfect for those who want to improve posture and build a stronger core.

Why it works:
Pilates enhances core strength, improves flexibility, and promotes balanced muscle development.

How to start:
Join a Pilates class or follow instructional videos online. Consistency is key, so aim for 2-3 sessions per week.

For Advanced: Pushing the Limits

For those who are already in great shape and looking for more intense workouts, advanced activities can provide the challenge needed to reach peak fitness levels.

High-Intensity Interval Training (HIIT)

HIIT involves short bursts of intense exercise followed by brief rest periods. It's highly effective for burning fat and improving cardiovascular fitness.

Why it works:

HIIT boosts metabolism, burns a significant number of calories in a short time, and improves athletic performance.

How to start:
Include HIIT sessions 2-3 times a week, combining exercises like sprinting, jumping jacks, and burpees.

Weightlifting
For those looking to build strength and muscle mass, weightlifting is the way to go. It involves lifting weights to target specific muscle groups.

Why it works:
Weightlifting increases muscle mass, boosts metabolic rate, and improves overall strength.

How to start:
Follow a structured weightlifting program, focusing on different muscle groups each session. Consider working with a trainer to ensure proper form and technique.

Advanced Yoga

For seasoned yogis, advanced yoga offers more challenging poses and deeper meditation practices. It's a holistic way to enhance physical and mental well-being.

<u>Why it works:</u>
Advanced yoga builds strength, flexibility, and mental clarity.

<u>How to start:</u>
Practise advanced poses like headstands, arm balances, and deep backbends. Consistent practice and guidance from a skilled instructor are recommended.

No matter your fitness level, there's a physical activity that can help you on your weight management journey. The key is to find exercises that you enjoy and that match your current abilities. By progressively challenging yourself and staying consistent, you'll not only achieve your weight goals but also improve your overall health and well-being.

Chapter 9: Long-Term Maintenance of Weight Loss

Strategies for Preventing Weight Regain

Congratulations, you've reached your weight loss goal! Now comes the critical part: maintaining your new, healthier weight. Many people find that keeping the weight off can be as challenging as losing it in the first place. Let's dive into some effective strategies for preventing weight regain and ensuring your hard-earned results last a lifetime.

Adopt a Sustainable Eating Plan

One of the most common pitfalls after weight loss is reverting to old eating habits. To prevent this, adopt a sustainable eating plan that you can maintain in the long term.

<u>Balanced Diet:</u>

Focus on a balanced diet rich in whole foods, including plenty of fruits, vegetables, lean proteins, and whole grains. Avoid extreme diets that are hard to stick to.

Portion Control:

Keep an eye on portion sizes to prevent overeating. Use smaller plates and be mindful of serving sizes.

Mindful Eating:

Practice mindful eating by paying attention to hunger and fullness cues. Eat slowly, savor your food, and avoid distractions like TV or smartphones during meals.

Stay Physically Active

Regular physical activity is crucial for weight maintenance. It not only helps you burn calories but also boosts your metabolism and improves overall health.

Consistent Routine:

Aim for at least 150 minutes of moderate-intensity exercise or 75 minutes of vigorous-intensity exercise per week. Incorporate a mix of cardio, strength training, and flexibility exercises.

Find Enjoyable Activities:

Choose physical activities that you enjoy, whether it's dancing, hiking, swimming, or cycling. When you enjoy what you're doing, you're more likely to stick with it.

<u>Stay Active Throughout the Day:</u>

Incorporate movement into your daily routine. Take the stairs instead of the elevator, walk or bike to work, and take regular breaks to stretch or walk around if you have a desk job.

Monitor Your Progress

Regularly monitoring your weight and other health metrics can help you stay on track and catch any potential weight regain early.

<u>Weigh Yourself:</u>

Weigh yourself regularly, but not obsessively. Weekly or bi-weekly weigh-ins can help you stay aware of any changes.

<u>Track Your Food:</u>

Keep a food journal or use a mobile app to track your meals and snacks. This can help you stay accountable and make healthier choices.

Check-in on Fitness:

Monitor your physical activity levels and progress in your fitness routine. Set new fitness goals to keep yourself motivated.

Manage Stress and Sleep

Stress and lack of sleep can negatively impact your weight by influencing your eating habits and hormone levels.

Stress Management:

Practice stress management techniques such as meditation, yoga, deep breathing exercises, or engaging in hobbies you enjoy.

Prioritize Sleep:

Aim for 7-9 hours of quality sleep per night. Establish a regular sleep schedule, create a calming bedtime routine, and ensure your sleep environment is conducive to rest.

Stay Hydrated

Drinking enough water is essential for overall health and can aid in weight maintenance.

Water Intake:

Aim to drink at least 8 cups (64 ounces) of water daily. Adjust your intake based on your activity level and climate.

Limit Sugary Drinks:

Avoid sugary drinks like soda, sweetened teas, and energy drinks, which can add unnecessary calories to your diet.

Build a Support System

Having a support system can make a significant difference in maintaining your weight loss.

Family and Friends:

Surround yourself with supportive family and friends who encourage your healthy lifestyle choices.

Join a Group:

Consider joining a weight maintenance group or online community where you can share experiences, get advice, and stay motivated.

<u>Professional Help:</u>

Don't hesitate to seek support from healthcare professionals such as dietitians, nutritionists, or therapists if you need extra guidance.

Keep Setting Goals

Setting new, non-weight-related goals can help you stay motivated and focused on maintaining a healthy lifestyle.

<u>Fitness Goals:</u>

Challenge yourself with new fitness goals, such as running a race, mastering a new yoga pose, or increasing your strength.

<u>Personal Growth:</u>

Set goals for personal growth, such as learning a new skill, starting a new hobby, or achieving a work-related milestone.

Maintaining weight loss is an ongoing journey that requires dedication and persistence. By adopting sustainable eating habits, staying active, monitoring your progress, managing stress and sleep, staying hydrated, building a support system, and continuously setting new goals, you can prevent weight regain and enjoy the benefits of a healthier lifestyle.

Support Systems and Resources for Continued Success

Maintaining your weight loss is a journey that requires ongoing support, resources, and motivation. Having a strong support system and access to helpful resources can make all the difference in staying on track and continuing to succeed. Let's explore how you can build a network of support and utilize available resources to maintain your healthy lifestyle for the long term.

Building Your Support System

A solid support system can provide encouragement, accountability, and motivation. Here are some ways to build and strengthen your network:

Family and Friends

Your closest allies are often those who know you best. Involve your family and friends in your journey to ensure you have a strong foundation of support.

Communicate Your Goals:

Share your weight maintenance goals with your loved ones. Let them know how they can support you, whether it's through joining you for workouts, preparing healthy meals together, or simply offering encouragement.

Engage in Activities Together:
Participate in physical activities with your family and friends. Whether it's hiking, biking, or taking a fitness class, being active together can be both fun and motivating.

Support Groups
Joining a support group can provide a sense of community and shared experience. There are various types of groups available, both in-person and online.

Weight Maintenance Groups:
Look for groups specifically focused on maintaining weight loss. These groups offer a platform to share challenges, successes, and strategies.

Fitness Communities:
Engage with local or online fitness communities where members encourage each other to stay active and healthy.

Professional Support

Sometimes, professional guidance is necessary to keep you on the right path. Don't hesitate to seek help from experts.

Dietitians and Nutritionists:

Consult with a registered dietitian or nutritionist for personalized advice and meal planning. They can help you navigate challenges and ensure your diet remains balanced.

Personal Trainers:

Work with a personal trainer to create a tailored fitness plan that evolves with your progress and keeps you motivated.

Therapists and Counselors:

If emotional or psychological factors are affecting your weight maintenance, a therapist or counselor can provide valuable support and strategies for coping.

Utilizing Available Resources

There are numerous resources available to help you stay informed, motivated, and on track. Here's a look at some useful tools and platforms:

Mobile Apps

Technology can be a great ally in your weight maintenance journey. There are many apps designed to help you track your progress and stay motivated.

Nutrition Apps:

Apps like MyFitnessPal and Lose It! allow you to track your food intake, monitor nutrients, and maintain a food diary.

Fitness Apps:

Apps like Fitbit, Strava, and Nike Training Club offer workout plans, track your physical activity, and provide fitness challenges to keep you engaged.

Mindfulness and Meditation Apps:

Apps like Headspace and Calm offer guided meditations and mindfulness exercises to help you manage stress and maintain mental well-being.

Online Communities

Engaging with online communities can provide inspiration, advice, and a sense of belonging.

Social Media Groups:

Join Facebook groups, Reddit communities, or other social media platforms dedicated to weight maintenance and healthy living.

Forums and Discussion Boards:

Participate in forums like those on SparkPeople or WeightWatchers, where you can ask questions, share experiences, and find support.

Educational Resources

Stay informed about the latest research and strategies for weight maintenance through books, articles, and podcasts.

Books:

Read books by experts in nutrition, fitness, and psychology to gain deeper insights and practical tips (like this book you are reading now).

Articles and Blogs:

Follow reputable health websites and blogs to stay updated on new findings and trends.

Podcasts:

Listen to podcasts focused on health, fitness, and weight maintenance for ongoing motivation and learning.

Practical Tips for Leveraging Support Systems and Resources

To make the most of your support systems and resources, consider these practical tips:

Set Regular Check-Ins

Schedule regular check-ins with your support network to stay accountable and address any challenges.

Family and Friends:

Have weekly or monthly check-ins with your loved ones to discuss your progress and any obstacles you're facing.

Support Groups:

Attend group meetings regularly, whether they're in-person or virtual, to stay connected and motivated.

Professionals:

Book periodic appointments with your dietitian, personal trainer, or therapist to ensure you're on track and to get personalized advice.

Stay Engaged

Keep yourself engaged and motivated by setting new goals and trying new activities.

Fitness Challenges:

Participate in fitness challenges or events to keep your exercise routine exciting and goal-oriented.

Learning Opportunities:

Continuously educate yourself about health and wellness by attending workshops, webinars, or reading new material.

Variety in Routine:

Switch up your workouts and meal plans to prevent boredom and keep things interesting.

Maintaining your weight loss is a lifelong journey, and having the right support systems and resources can make it a fulfilling and sustainable one. By building a strong network of family, friends, support groups, and professionals, and by utilizing helpful tools and educational resources, you can stay motivated and equipped to handle any challenges that come your way.

Chapter 10: Myths and Facts about Obesity

Debunking Common Myths

When it comes to obesity, misinformation abounds. Misleading myths can lead to misunderstandings, stigma, and ineffective weight management strategies. Let's debunk some of the most common myths about obesity and set the record straight with evidence-based facts.

Myth 1: Obesity Is Just About Willpower

The Myth:

"If people had more self-control, they wouldn't be obese."

The Fact:

Obesity is a complex condition influenced by various factors, including genetics, environment, and biology. While personal choices play a role, they are not the sole determinants of body weight.

Myth 2: All Calories Are Equal

The Myth:

"A calorie is a calorie, no matter where it comes from."

The Fact:

Not all calories are created equal. The source of calories can impact how your body processes and stores them.

Myth 3: Dieting Is the Best Way to Lose Weight

The Myth:

"To lose weight, you just need to go on a diet."

The Fact:

Fad diets and extreme restrictions are not sustainable long-term solutions and can often lead to weight regain.

Myth 4: You Can't Be Overweight and Healthy

The Myth:

"All overweight people are unhealthy."

<u>The Fact:</u>

It's possible to be overweight and still be in good health, just as it's possible to be at a "normal" weight and have health problems.

Myth 5: Exercise Is Enough to Lose Weight

<u>The Myth:</u>

"You can out-exercise a bad diet."

<u>The Fact:</u>

While exercise is crucial for overall health and weight maintenance, it's difficult to achieve weight loss through exercise alone without dietary changes.

Myth 6: Carbs Are the Enemy

<u>The Myth:</u>

"All carbs are bad and should be avoided."

<u>The Fact:</u>

Carbohydrates are a necessary macronutrient and provide the body with energy. The key is choosing the right kinds of carbs.

Myth 7: Losing Weight Quickly Is the Best Way

<u>The Myth:</u>

"The faster you lose weight, the better."

<u>The Fact:</u>

Rapid weight loss can lead to muscle loss, nutritional deficiencies, and a higher likelihood of regaining weight.

Understanding the facts about obesity helps dispel myths and reduces stigma. By embracing a holistic view that considers genetics, environment, and biology, we can approach weight management with empathy and effectiveness.

Some Important Facts about Obesity

Gaining a true understanding of obesity requires sifting through a lot of information, some of which can be misleading. Let's explore some critical facts about obesity to debunk myths and illuminate this complex condition.

Fact 1: Obesity Is Multifaceted

Obesity isn't just about overeating or lack of exercise. It's a condition influenced by a combination of genetic, environmental, and psychological factors. They include:

Genetic Influence:

Your genetic makeup can significantly affect your body weight and fat storage. Genetics can influence appetite, metabolism, and fat distribution.

Environmental Factors:

Your surroundings impact your lifestyle choices, including access to healthy foods and safe exercise spaces, along with socioeconomic influences.

Psychological Aspects:

Emotional factors like stress and depression can also affect eating habits and physical activity levels.

Fact 2: Obesity Heightens the Risk of Many Diseases

Carrying excess weight increases the likelihood of developing numerous health conditions. Some of these conditions include:

Cardiovascular Disease:

Obesity is a major contributor to heart disease due to its effects on blood pressure, cholesterol, and inflammation.

Type 2 Diabetes:

There's a strong link between obesity and insulin resistance, which can lead to type 2 diabetes.

Certain Cancers:

Being overweight is associated with higher risks of cancers like breast, colon, and endometrial cancer.

Fact 3: Small Weight Loss Yields Big Health Benefits

You don't need to hit an ideal weight to reap health benefits. Losing even 5-10% of your body weight can make a significant difference. Some of the benefits are:

Blood Pressure Reduction:

Modest weight loss can help lower blood pressure.

Improved Cholesterol Levels:

It can also improve cholesterol, reducing the risk of heart disease.

Better Blood Sugar Control:

Weight loss can enhance blood sugar management, reducing the risk or helping manage type 2 diabetes.

Fact 4: Obesity Is a Global Issue

Obesity affects people worldwide, not just in wealthy nations. Some causes include:

Urbanization's Role:

Increased urban living leads to more sedentary lifestyles and greater access to high-calorie foods, contributing to rising obesity rates globally.

Dietary Shifts:

Many developing countries are moving from traditional diets to processed foods high in sugars and fats, fueling obesity.

Fact 5: Exercise Alone Isn't Enough

While exercise is essential for health and weight maintenance, it's usually insufficient on its own for substantial weight loss. Other activities should be considered including:

<u>Balancing Calories:</u>
Effective weight loss requires a calorie deficit, achieved through dietary changes and physical activity.

<u>Sustainable Practices:</u>
Long-term weight management relies on sustainable changes in both diet and exercise habits.

Fact 6: Stigma and Discrimination Are Pervasive
People with obesity often face stigma and discrimination, which can severely impact their mental and physical health. Some of the impacts include:

<u>Mental Health Impact:</u>
Weight stigma can lead to low self-esteem, depression, and anxiety.

<u>Healthcare Bias:</u>
Stigma can also result in biased treatment from healthcare providers, leading to inadequate care and worse health outcomes.

Fact 7: Early Prevention and Intervention Are Essential

Preventing obesity from a young age and addressing weight gain early are crucial. Some of the strategies involved include?

<u>Healthy Habits Early:</u>

Promoting healthy eating and regular physical activity from childhood can help prevent obesity.

<u>Community Support:</u>

Public health policies and community-based programs can support healthier environments and lifestyles.

By shedding light on these important facts, we can better understand the realities of obesity, empowering individuals and communities to take positive steps toward improved health. Knowledge is a powerful tool for driving meaningful change.

Chapter 11: Conclusion

Looking Ahead: Future Trends in Diet and Obesity Management

Personalised Nutrition

The Future

The days of one-size-fits-all diets are fading. Personalised nutrition, tailored to individual genetic, metabolic, and lifestyle factors, is gaining traction.

Genetic Insights

Genetic testing is advancing, offering insights into how our bodies respond to different foods, paving the way for customised diets that optimise health.

Metabolic Analysis

Understanding individual metabolic profiles can lead to more effective dietary recommendations.

Behavioural Customization

Tailoring interventions based on individual behaviours and preferences can enhance their success.

Digital Health Innovations

The Future

Technology is transforming diet and obesity management, making tracking progress and staying motivated easier than ever.

Apps and Wearables

Health apps and wearable devices provide real-time feedback on physical activity, calorie intake, and sleep patterns, empowering informed decisions.

Telehealth Services

Virtual consultations with dietitians and healthcare providers offer convenient, personalised guidance.

AI Tools

Artificial intelligence can analyse vast data to provide personalised dietary advice, predict health outcomes, and identify risks.

Functional Foods and Nutraceuticals

The Future

The food industry is innovating with functional foods and nutraceuticals aimed at promoting health and managing weight.

Probiotics and Prebiotics

These gut-friendly compounds are recognized for their role in improving digestion, enhancing metabolism, and supporting weight management.

Plant-Based Options

The rise of plant-based diets and meat substitutes provides healthier, sustainable eating options.

Bioactive Ingredients

Foods enriched with bioactive compounds, like antioxidants and anti-inflammatory agents, are being developed to support overall health and weight management.

Psychological and Behavioural Approaches

The Future

Addressing the psychological aspects of eating is becoming essential in obesity management.

Mindful Eating

Mindfulness practices, such as mindful eating, are being integrated into weight management programs to foster a healthier relationship with food.

Cognitive Behavioral Therapy (CBT)

CBT addresses emotional eating and other behaviours contributing to obesity, offering tools for lasting change.

Stress Reduction

Stress management and emotional well-being programs are becoming integral to comprehensive obesity management.

The Future

Public health initiatives and community programs are evolving to create environments that support healthy lifestyles.

Policy Initiatives

Governments are enacting policies to reduce unhealthy food availability and promote nutritious options, such as taxing sugary drinks and subsidising fruits and vegetables.

Local Programs

Community initiatives, like gardens, fitness classes, and nutrition workshops, are empowering healthier choices.

School Interventions

Programs targeting children and adolescents focus on establishing healthy habits early, with schools playing a pivotal role in obesity prevention.

The Future

A holistic approach to health is emerging, recognizing the interconnectedness of physical, mental, and emotional well-being.

Integrated Care Models

Healthcare systems are moving towards models that address all aspects of health, including diet, exercise, mental health, and social factors.

Preventive Focus

Emphasis is shifting towards preventive care, maintaining health through lifestyle choices and early interventions.

Health at Every Size (HAES)

The HAES movement promotes body positivity and health improvements regardless of weight, reducing stigma and fostering a more inclusive health approach.

As we continue to evolve and refine our strategies, embracing these innovations and maintaining a commitment to holistic, individualised, and compassionate care will be key to success. By staying informed and open to new possibilities, we can work towards a healthier future for everyone.

Appendix: Resources and Further Reading

Glossary of Terms

Basal Metabolic Rate (BMR)

The number of calories per day, your body requires to maintain essential physiological functions at rest.

Body Mass Index (BMI)

A measure of body fat based on height and weight, used to classify individuals into different weight categories.

Calories

Units of energy provided by food and drinks. 1 calorie equals 4.2 joules

Carbohydrates

One of the three main macronutrients, serving as the primary energy source for the body.

Dietary Fiber

A type of carbohydrate that the body can't digest, but is helpful in improving bowel movement and preventing constipation. Found in fruits, vegetables, whole grains, and legumes.

Insulin Resistance

A condition where the body's cells become less responsive to insulin, often resulting in higher blood glucose levels. This is usually seen in type 2 diabetes.

Macronutrients

Nutrients needed in larger amounts that provide energy and raw materials for body building i.e carbohydrates, proteins, and fats.

Metabolism

Refers to all chemical reactions and processes within a living organism that maintain life, including the conversion of food into energy.

Obesity

A medical condition characterised by excessive body fat, increasing the risk of health issues.

Proteins

One of the three main macronutrients, crucial for building and repairing tissues, and for making enzymes and hormones.

Saturated Fats

A type of fat found in animal products and certain oils, which can elevate cholesterol levels.

Type 2 Diabetes

A chronic condition that affects how the body processes blood sugar (glucose). Usually associated with Obesity

Recommended Websites and Other Books

Some excellent websites to get more information!

Academy of Nutrition and Dietetics (eatright.org)

Description:

This site provides science-based advice on nutrition, health, and fitness, featuring dietary guidelines, meal planning tips, and recipes.

Why It's Helpful:

Whether you're making dietary adjustments or seeking specific nutrition information, you'll find expert guidance here.

Centers for Disease Control and Prevention (cdc.gov/healthyweight)

Description:

The CDC offers extensive resources on achieving and maintaining a healthy weight, covering topics like obesity, physical activity, and weight loss strategies.

Why It's Helpful:

It's your go-to for the latest health data and evidence-based weight management strategies.

National Institute of Diabetes and Digestive and Kidney Diseases (niddk.nih.gov)

Description:

This site provides comprehensive information on obesity, including causes, health consequences, and treatment options.

Why It's Helpful:

Ideal for in-depth research and understanding obesity-related health issues from a scientific viewpoint.

MyPlate (<u>myplate.gov</u>)

<u>Description:</u>

Managed by the U.S. Department of Agriculture, MyPlate offers practical information to help you create a healthier diet using a simple plate graphic.

<u>Why It's Helpful:</u>

Perfect for visual learners who appreciate clear, straightforward advice on portion control and balanced meals.

Harvard T.H. Chan School of Public Health (<u>hsph.harvard.edu/nutritionsource</u>)

<u>Description:</u>

The Nutrition Source is packed with information on healthy eating, debunking common myths, and exploring the latest nutrition research.

<u>Why It's Helpful:</u>

Great for those who want to stay updated on the latest scientific findings in nutrition.

"The Obesity Code: Unlocking the Secrets of Weight Loss" by Dr. Jason Fung

<u>Description:</u>

Dr. Fung explores the hormonal causes of weight gain and suggests strategies for managing insulin to achieve sustainable weight loss.

<u>Why It's Helpful:</u>

This book offers a fresh take on weight loss, moving beyond conventional calorie-counting methods.

"Intuitive Eating: A Revolutionary Anti-Diet Approach" by Evelyn Tribole and Elyse Resch

<u>Description:</u>

This book introduces intuitive eating, encouraging readers to listen to their body's hunger and fullness signals rather than following diets.

It promotes a compassionate approach to eating, aimed at fostering a healthy relationship with food.

"Why We Get Fat: And What to Do About It" by Gary Taubes

Description:

Taubes delves into the science of obesity, challenging common beliefs about diet and fat.

Why It's Helpful:

For those interested in the science behind obesity and diet, this book provides a thorough and engaging analysis.

"The Complete Guide to Fasting: Heal Your Body Through Intermittent, Alternate-Day, and Extended Fasting" by Dr. Jason Fung and Jimmy Moore

<u>Description:</u>

This guide explores various fasting methods and their benefits for weight loss and overall health.

<u>Why It's Helpful:</u>

It's a comprehensive resource for anyone interested in incorporating fasting into their lifestyle.

"Food Rules: An Eater's Manual" by Michael Pollan

<u>Description:</u>

Pollan offers simple, memorable rules for healthy eating, distilled from his extensive research into food and diet.

<u>Why It's Helpful:</u>

This book provides straightforward, actionable advice that's easy to remember and apply to everyday eating habits.

THANKS FOR READING!